Dr. Charles "Chod" DeLong is a psychiatrist who practiced psychoanalytically oriented psychotherapy for 35 years. After he retired, he asked himself what one thing he had learned in his practice that would help the human race to evolve emotionally. He spent the next five years reviewing his patients and looking for common threads and themes. The answer he ultimately arrived at, "Personal Integrity," is the inspiration for this book.

T0165432

In this short book, veteran psychiatrist Dr. Chod DeLong guides us through a process of "active understanding." Using numerous case studies to illustrate his point, he shows us how "active understanding" works and why he believes it is the highest form of kindness that we can give to ourselves as well as to others. I use the wisdom in this book each day. Achieving Personal Integrity may forever change your life for the better.

Judy Block
Former Articles Editor, Psychology Today

For more information and to share how *Achieving Personal Integrity* has affected you, please visit:
www.achievingpersonalintegrity.com

Achieving Personal Integrity: A Psychiatrist's Insights

Charles C. DeLong, MD

iUniverse, Inc.
Bloomington

Achieving Personal Integrity:
A Psychiatrist's Insights

The information, ideas, and suggestions in this book are not intended as a substitute for professional medical advice. Before following any suggestions contained in this book, you should consult your personal physician. Neither the author nor the publisher shall be liable or responsible for any loss or damage allegedly arising as a consequence of your use or application of any information or suggestions in this book.

iUniverse books may be ordered through booksellers or by contacting:

iUniverse
1663 Liberty Drive
Bloomington, IN 47403
www.iuniverse.com
1-800-Authors (1-800-288-4677)

Because of the dynamic nature of the Internet, any web addresses or links contained in this book may have changed since publication and may no longer be valid. The views expressed in this work are solely those of the author and do not necessarily reflect the views of the publisher, and the publisher hereby disclaims any responsibility for them.

ISBN: 978-1-4759-2862-4 (sc)
ISBN: 978-1-4759-2863-1 (hc)
ISBN: 978-1-4759-2864-8 (e)

Library of Congress Control Number: 2012909145

Printed in the United States of America

iUniverse rev. date: 06/06/2012

Dedicated to the memory of
Maurice Levine, M.D.
Chairman Department of Psychiatry
University of Cincinnati
Cincinnati, Ohio
1947-1974

Table of Contents

Introduction

S ometime during my freshman year in college I decided to become a psychiatrist. Looking back, it was probably because I'd always been more comfortable observing, rather than wholeheartedly participating in, group affairs. As far back as grade school, even while in the sandbox, I can remember hearing the grown-ups on the porch talking about "Why people act the way they do."

I enjoyed medical school and a rotating internship despite the fact that they were quite demanding. I was fortunate to get into a top psychiatric residency program at the University of Cincinnati. As I look back upon my residency, even then I was developing an awareness and appreciation for what the patient was actively trying to resolve regardless of his or her diagnosis. Next came two years of active duty in the Naval Reserve as a hospital psychiatrist in Bremerton, Washington, and then Camp Pendleton, California.

I entered private practice in 1968 in Palo Alto, California. For the first 20 years or so I had an active hospital practice in addition to conducting 40 hours a week of outpatient psychotherapy in my office. In the beginning of my practice, with each patient, I waited for "transference" to develop, the process wherein the patient begins to bring their emotional problems into our relationship and to work them out. While this process seemed to work eventually, I began to notice that from day one each patient was actively trying to resolve their emotional conflicts and evolve their personalities long before any transference was evident. This process of resolving and evolving seemed to go much faster if I, as their therapist, was more comfortable with their attempts to do so then they were themselves. The more calm and connected I remained, the more progress I saw in them, a process known as "active understanding" and the key ingredient to successfully living with personal integrity.

Early in my practice I underwent psychoanalysis myself for more than seven years, and eventually retired after three decades.

In January of 2010 I was diagnosed with multiple myeloma, a cancer of the bone marrow. This resulted in a great deal of pain, a total disruption of my daily living due to various therapies, counting out pills, and doctors visits, as well as a great assault on my mind thanks to chemotherapies that are characterized by pain, exhaustion, and "my brain just doesn't do what it used to do."

Attempting to write this book, despite the fact that I had some pretty well-thought-out notes, has been the hardest thing I have ever tried to do. Not just because I was attempting to write my first book at age 74, and not just because I was in pain and exhausted, but because of the direct effect of the chemotherapy. Well, I'm writing the book the best I can with the idea that somebody else may have to revise it for me, as there may be no tomorrow. While the book may not be well-written, I do feel that the message about active understanding and living with personal integrity is a good one.

In my private practice, I did mainly psychotherapy as opposed to psychopharmacology. I worked one-on-one with my patients rather than prescribing pills. Over the years, I learned much about how to resolve emotional conflicts and understand anger to eventually live with personal integrity. This book is a guide for developing your own personality with integrity, which, as you will see, can have a profound effect on your interpersonal relationships. The book includes theory, how-to steps, and examples.

It is the purpose of this book to make this process of becoming a personality with integrity explicit, in the hope that you will become skillful in this endeavor and reap the benefits, so the whole process will become self-reinforcing and eventually practiced by all in our society. I believe this will result in our attaining new levels of freedom, security, mutuality, appreciation for the other, and the ability to help each other. That is, the human race can now resume its evolution.

NOTE: Many of the examples included here were drawn from actual cases. Names and details have been changed to protect confidentiality.

Chapter 1:

———•◆•———

What is Personal Integrity?

B efore we can learn *how* to live with personal integrity, it's important to understand the attributes that people with personal integrity share. First and foremost, people with personal integrity are entirely comfortable with themselves and with their feelings, so much so that they do not require support from the environment. By support from the environment we mean external validation, such as approval or guaranteed acceptance. They can accept criticism, rejection, even hostility. They don't take things personally or regress emotionally into the sensitivities of their own unresolved emotional conflicts.

Let's look at an example of how someone with personal integrity reacts to an unpleasant, even hostile, remark.

At a potluck supper, "Susan" who always brings generous amounts of elaborate dishes, sharply criticizes "Ellen" for bringing a skimpy amount of a rather plain dish. Ellen accepts Susan's criticism comfortably as an accurate reflection of both how Susan assessed things and felt about the situation and as a possibly legitimate, and perhaps even accurate, commentary on her own contributions. She was not at all hurt and remained available for more of Susan's opinions and comments. When Ellen acknowledged the paucity and plainness of her dishes, Susan went on further to say "I wouldn't dare to offer what you bring." Instead of responding with anger, hurt or retaliation, Ellen, knowing this slight is not personal, looked at the situation from Susan's point of view and responded, "I know, I think you're afraid of what people will think so you won't risk bringing anything but the very best. This is probably why you require so much of yourself." By adhering to her personal integrity, Ellen completely disarms Susan and puts her in touch with the source of her frustration. Susan replies, "You know, I think you're right! And when I see that you are so at ease with yourself, and that I have to be so hard on myself, it really makes me angry!" This was said with a smile and a twinkle in her eye. We could guess that their relationship will now be based on greater mutual confidence and respect.

Ellen, who has a personality with integrity, is not at the mercy of the environment for emotional support, which includes Susan's opinion of her, and is able to stay in the "here-and-now" external reality. This is adaptive because it allows Ellen to objectively stay in the relationship with Susan and not become immersed in her own feelings. A personality without integrity is dependent upon the environment for support of their emotions, as Susan in the above example worried about what others thought of her, and, therefore lashed out at Ellen. This significantly compromises adaptability.

Personalities with integrity, like Ellen's, have the capacity to "get beyond themselves" and stay there long enough to perceive and understand reality. Too often we become mired in our not-so-well-understood emotional conflicts and don't perceive and understand reality enough to get the overall picture. Another trait shared by people with personal integrity is their ability to recognize frustration. In moments of potential frustration, they are aware that the world isn't providing according to their wishes, they accept this, and recalibrate their expectations to line up with reality. Their wish likely will continue to exist but the anger about this wish subsides when the fact that it will not be gratified is accepted. They may subsequently have to deal with the disappointment of the personal loss, but this is a separate problem, involving their degree of emotional investment in the thing that was lost. Again, there are two parts to this: first, anger over the fact that the wish will not be gratified and the dissipation of this anger when this expectation is renounced and, second, sorrow and disappointment stemming from the lack of gratification of the wish which will not disappear until the wish subsides.

Let's look at an example of how a personality with integrity deals with frustration. If my three–year-old daughter dies, at first I am both angry and sad. Eventually, when I accept the fact that she's never coming back, my anger subsides; I accept that my wish to have her back will not be gratified. However, even though I have accepted reality, my wish to have her will continue and I will continue to feel sad. The sadness will remain until the wish subsides. This may involve the process of mourning, of denial, or the gratification of a similar wish such as having another child. An "unevolved" personality tends to just become angry, incapable of identifying their own unrealistic expectations, and consequently unable to align their expectations with reality. Their frustration and anger will continue unabated.

Further traits you will notice shared by those with personal integrity are that they tend to be comfortable with themselves as well as others, and the world in general. They approach just about every interaction with *active understanding*; a concept which will be further explained in Chapter 3. They have a pleasant self-confidence and the capacity to enjoy their activities, others, and the world without judgment. They tend to be accepting of their own anger and to regard it as a signal that their expectations are unrealistic and in need of recalibration, thereby tending to have less anger, and to never discharge their anger outside of the verbal arena. We will discuss anger and its root causes in Chapter 2.

You will notice that when those with personal integrity attempt to evolve, the changes will tend to be subtle and not so dramatic. On the other hand, a person who has not yet achieved personal integrity will struggle because they lack the techniques to move themselves forward, which leads to recurrent failures to evolve their maturational arrests, meaning that they must start at whatever primitive level at which they got "stuck" and then attempt to evolve from there. Their attempts can be quite challenging and require understanding from those around them because they often unknowingly set up situations that accommodate their primitive techniques in order to try to advance. They will try to set up situations where they can experience the full depth of these immature feelings. In attempting to do so they may project anger or criticism upon others and thereby experience this as an attack from outside themselves. For example, "Kathy's" parents were hostile, critical and controlling. Kathy grew up fearful of herself and of her parents and tried to hide herself from them. She was inhibited, quiet, anxious and wary, if not frightened, of herself. She imagined that others would find her objectionable and often misinterpreted remarks about her as criticism. She tended to keep people back and away from her with low-grade hostile sarcastic remarks. She never risked expressing her feelings, her new ideas or playfulness.

Kathy became a member of a group of women who hiked for three or four miles at a time twice a week. The conversations tended to be pleasant and somewhat superficial. She listened intently, found the other women's personal accounts of their feelings and experiences meaningful, but could never venture hers. One day while walking, without any apparent provocation, she began to express herself. Angrily, she accused the group of mistreating her with hostility, criticism and control. All of the members were surprised and some were shocked. This was the first time that she had ever risked expressing her feelings and it resulted in a distancing from many of the other women. As a result, she started walking more with just one member named "Roberta". As they walked they discussed her outburst with the group. Kathy reiterated her grievances and Roberta just listened. Roberta comfortably accepted Kathy's complaints and discussed them with her at length. Roberta eventually indicated that while she didn't feel that Kathy's issues were well founded she did feel that Kathy's perceptions and/or misperceptions were quite worthy of taking seriously and of being understood. During their subsequent walks, Kathy began to risk expression of her feelings with Roberta. It was very difficult for her because her inner self was so infused with anger, but they both seemed to realize that it was the best she could do. After particularly abrasive moments Roberta would keep the conversation going, unlike others who would turn away. At times Roberta would say with a pleasant look on her face "a little more gently, please." Here, Kathy is reconnecting to herself as she was in her early childhood and trying to evolve from there. This meant that she had to reconnect with the horror of those years. She had to risk being her real self, for better or worse, and evolve from there. This involved the pain that was inflicted upon her, her painfully low self-esteem, her rage and her inability to play, to enjoy and to be optimistic. On her walks with Roberta she began to risk more than she ever had before with another human being. She was beginning to grow emotionally by learning to accept and understand her troublesome feelings. This was mainly because of Roberta's comfort level with her anger.

During one of their walks Kathy suddenly burst into tears and exclaimed "I want to be your friend, but I have nothing to offer." Roberta replied "You bring your real self, for better or worse, to our relationship and that's more than any of the other gals do." With Kathy, Roberta got a meaningful connection. Interestingly, Kathy's expression of anger when she was with the group, except for that one time, was only to maintain some distance from the others and didn't involve risking her real feelings.

Later, in her walks with Roberta she began to risk connecting to her real feelings, as uncomfortable as they were. Thanks to

Roberta's comfortable acceptance she was able to come to grips with these troublesome feelings and grow emotionally in ways that were not possible in childhood with her primitive parents. It's much easier to be comfortable with Kathy's anger when one realizes that its expression is in the service of her emotional growth and personality evolution.

Personalities with integrity help other people by accepting parts of them that they cannot accept which may include anger, conflict, negative self-esteem and even sadness. I recall a patient who had sobbed about her sadness throughout a three-year period in therapy. Several years later toward the end of her sessions with me, she reflected on this time with the remark, "You (doctor) stayed connected to me all those years when I cried and cried!" It was during this time that she came to grips with the grief of her terribly sad childhood and eventually her depressions disappeared. The important thing here is that as her therapist I stayed absolutely comfortable and connected to her while she sobbed for two or three hours a week for three years. Of course it's much easier in my role as a therapist to avoid taking anything personally or distorting reality but the principle is the same.

The ultimate example of personal integrity occurs in those who are able to comfortably accept any and all of their own and other people's feelings. They view others just as they are because they have no need to distort their perception of the real world according to their own needs, conflicts or unrelated feelings. In short, they do not need to use others or the environment to maintain their equanimity. People without personal integrity are frequently engulfed by their feelings stemming from unresolved conflicts and, as a result, leave the here-and-now external reality and lose that sense of calm and self-control.

Let's look at another example of a situation involving a person with integrity: a father is dining out with his twenty-year-old daughter. In the midst of their conversation, she suddenly says, "You're a terrible father." He asks, "How's that?" She replies, "You should know, we've been over this many times before, and I'm not going to tell you again." The father nods, accepting this possibility, obviously comfortable with his daughter's opinion and appreciating the risk she might be taking by bringing her real self, for better or worse, into the trusted relationship with him. The subject changed for a while but then she said, "I have this problem. I'm spending too much of my time with Jack in Los Angeles and not enough time with Bob in Seattle. If you weren't such an insensitive father I wouldn't have this problem." She didn't elaborate and let the conversation lapse. Her father waited patiently. She then broke the silence with "I guess I'll have to start going to Seattle!" This was said with a sense of conclusion. She then seemed satisfied, became calmer, and didn't bring up the issue again.

While we don't know what was motivating her comments, what is clear is her father's comfort level with her and her opinions. While the father may not have fully understood his daughter's internal struggle, certainly in the beginning, he was nevertheless at ease with her opinion as to his perceived "terrible (ness)" and "insensitivity." We could suspect that the father's relaxed tone was helpful to his troubled daughter as she solved her problem. The father demonstrated the integrity of his personality by his ability to stay calmly focused on his daughter and her struggle. By staying in the understanding mode he was not available to take his daughter's derogatory accusations personally; he wasn't dependent upon the environment, in this case, his daughter's opinion of him, to support his self-image, nor in any way apparently dependent upon it. This was accomplished not by avoiding the environment or denying the criticism, but by his understanding. He was fully aware and accepting of the environment. He did not have to exclude any aspect of it by denial or avoidance. Interestingly, if he can do this, maybe his daughter can, too and eventually resolve her conflict. And, someday she may even start handling reality the way her father does.

Now, let's look at what we see so often: the father displaying a lack of personal integrity in his response. In this version, the father reacts to "you're a terrible father" with hurt: "You can't talk to me this way," and "I buy you a nice meal and you insult me." Here, he's completely at the mercy of the environment to support his self-esteem. He doesn't feel comfortable enough with himself to withstand the external criticism. He experiences emotional discomfort, and in all probability sees his daughter as the source of his unrest. The source of his unrest is actually his own deep-seated poor self-image, which his daughter's comments mobilized. Here he has left the external reality and the understanding that it might afford. And, he has regressed emotionally into the discomfort of his less-than-adequate self-image.

As this example demonstrates, a lack of personal integrity puts one at the mercy of the environment, further understanding is precluded, adaptation to the environment stops, and frequently both parties suffer.

Here's another example. "Mark" and "Sarah" are a very mature married couple. Mark tells Sarah what he would like to do on Saturday afternoon. Sarah responds by telling Mark exactly *how his activity will impact her*. Sarah's remark, even if it is unfavorable, is both gracious and responsible as it permits Mark to make the final decision based on both of their needs. However, so often when one's wishes are met by their partner's reluctance, annoyance, irritation, or anger the mutual understanding process screeches to a halt. In this case, Mark was very comfortable with his needs and, therefore, able to welcome Sarah's response whatever it might be. Mark's desire to gratify his wish/need is entirely separate from his spouse's level of comfort with it.

Personalities with integrity, whenever hurt or angered by the environment, ask themselves "what is it I can't accept?" They let themselves feel their discomfort, begin to identify the cause, and then recalibrate their expectations of their wish gratification to be in sync with reality.

Obviously, nobody's perfect. There will be times in an encounter that we may become irritated or downright angry. As our integrity develops, hopefully we can begin to recognize this, not become immediately engulfed in it, and put it aside to be dealt with later as one of our own unresolved emotional conflicts needing attention. And, hopefully, either retain our focus on the here-and-now external environment or immediately return to it.

To sum up, personal integrity means that we can understand, accept, and deal as facilitatively as possible with our feelings to the extent that we do not turn to the environment for help. That is, we are not dependent emotionally upon the environment. And, moreover, we are not available to exploit others in relationships. Our view of reality is not compromised. When we are unable to resolve our emotional problems, that is understand and accept our thoughts and feelings, we are subject at any time to becoming immersed in them.

Now that we know what comprises personal integrity, let's look at some of the things that get in the way of achieving it.

Chapter 2:

---•◆•---

What Stands in the Way of Achieving Personal Integrity

Before we can learn how to become a personality with integrity, we must understand the roadblocks that can impede our journey and some of the basic traits that we human beings share. In this chapter, we will look at accepting reality, anger, the thrust to grow, nature and nurture and narcissism.

Part 1: Reality

Understanding our world and the people in it, the "external reality", for what they are greatly increases our adaptability. The best relationships are those in which each party accepts the other just as they are, for better or worse. Obviously, these relationships must start with people who are willing to risk exposure of their real self. On the contrary, think how much a relationship would be limited by somebody unwilling to risk personal exposure, as in *"if you can't say something nice, don't say anything."* Not much meaningful could happen in those circumstances.

By "external reality," used above, we mean primarily the present reality of the relationship and the immediate environment as opposed to one's internal feelings and thoughts. The external reality would include the exact conversation, the presentation of the other person, and the immediate physical setting. These are in contrast to and distinct from what might be happening inside of us emotionally, our "internal reality." This most commonly occurs by our emotionally reliving some troublesome feelings that have absolutely nothing to do directly with the present external reality. For example, "Brian" is about to catch a flight at the airport. He enters the x-ray machine, stands with his hands above his head and the machine appears to have done its thing. As Brian starts to walk off over the big yellow footprints to retrieve his bags, the attendant says "Stop" and steps forward with his hands up as if to block Brian's body. Brian feels rage and thinks *"Who are you to order me around, to control me, to physically constrain me?"* and begins to experience all his previous resentment about being controlled and abused. At this point, Brian has completely left the "external reality" and regressed into his unresolved emotional conflicts about control and abuse. The attendant then says "Okay, you can go through now, the machine says you're clear." With this, Brian begins to return to the here and now reality of getting his bags, tying his shoes, and finding his gate.

As the above example illustrates, how we perceive reality and how we treat it is often determined by our negative feelings. Our unresolved conflicts stem from our inability to accept certain feelings and aspects of ourselves. Normally we try to avoid our feelings of discomfort by keeping them out of our awareness – out of our reality. This happens all by itself. In psychological terms, we automatically tend to *repress* uncomfortable feelings by pushing them outside of our awareness and keeping them there.

When our unresolved emotional conflicts enter the picture, our interpretation of reality is no longer based on any kind of objective observation. Effecting a facilitative solution is now out of the question. More important is the fact that we are not entirely in touch with the present reality and are trying to use the environment to meet our emotional needs regardless of how inappropriate the environment may be. In addition, we are confusing our internal conflicts with the external environment. This is a huge price that people without integrity pay.

The thing that most commonly interferes with our ability to stay in reality and its subsequent perception is our tendency to take things personally. So often a troubled acquaintance tries to tell us as best they can about their plight. They are angry. They may verbally attack us or blame us for their woes. A common response is discomfort, withdrawal within a troubled part of us, and/or maligning them. Once we develop the skills to live with personal integrity, we can avoid these automatic responses and stay in reality. Too often we become mired in our own not-so-well-understood emotional conflicts and don't perceive and understand reality enough to get the overall picture.

Reconciling ourselves with reality is accomplished by immersing ourselves in our own anger, feeling it as fully as possible, and then identifying our wishes that are not being gratified and renouncing our expectation that the world will gratify them. If we are unable to accept the fact that reality will not gratify our wishes, we experience anger. This can interfere with our perception of the external environment in a number of ways. People who are intent upon avoiding experiencing anger, that is, keeping their anger out of awareness, will selectively steer clear of aspects of the world (reality) that might give rise to anger. Moreover, they may be drawn to just "safe" things or events, thus limiting their perspective. Another person might focus on finding targets in the external world that would justify their maligning or discharging their anger upon the other either verbally or physically.

It is important to keep in mind the distinction between the acceptance of a wish and the gratification of a wish. Let's use a simple example of a hostile comment made by a friend. Our *acceptance* of their wish to hurt us is simply our comfort with their angry statement, the associated wish, and their attempt to make us uncomfortable. *Gratification* of their wish would be our responding with any kind of discomfort, anger, or hurt.

Interestingly, it is entirely possible for the angry would-be-perpetrator to be so uncomfortable with their wish to hurt us that they themselves reject their wish and, at the same time, make attempts to gratify it by making us uncomfortable or hurting us. Their rejection of the wish is based on their discomfort with it rather than on their understanding of it and their eventual acceptance and resolution of it. This often happens when somebody strongly wants something but doesn't feel that they deserve it. They may look to gratify the wish in situations where it cannot be gratified or unwittingly sabotage its gratification. Many people have a great deal of ambivalence about their wishes and/or their attempts to gratify them.

For example, "Joe" is a competent, hard-working electrician. He wants a promotion to foreman, has been up for it before but never gotten it, and is very bitter about it. Joe has a conflict. While he wants this promotion very much and, by the usual standards deserves it, he has trouble accepting it. Joe has always had low self-esteem and therefore would not risk much, e.g., jumping into a leadership role. He has had an attitude of not-deserving since childhood and has never been able to easily accept anything nice that comes his way. He is also self-conscious and not comfortable being the head of a group, entering a home to render an estimate, or generally taking charge. He isn't always well organized. So, while part of Joe wants the promotion and feels that he deserves it, that is, wants gratification of this wish, there is another part of Joe that cannot accept or allow gratification of this wish. This internal conflict is played out on the job at times when a foreman is not being sought by vehement requests for promotion, angry complaints of not being appreciated, repeated attempts to make his boss feel guilty about not promoting him, and arduous efforts to please the boss by doing extra work. This is the part of Joe that is seeking gratification of the wish for a promotion. At other times, when a new foreman is being sought and Joe is considered, he becomes anxious and withdrawn and generally sabotages his chances of promotion by being rude and uncommunicative to his boss, making mistakes, coming in late, etc. This is the part of Joe that cannot comfortably accept gratification of his wish for a promotion and thereby self-sabotages. In all probability, Joe experiences this problem as a conflict between himself and his workplace. He probably has little or no awareness that the basis for this problem is a conflict that is entirely internal and has nothing to do with the external environment. If Joe could

21

experience this conflict as his own he would have a better chance of coming to grips with it. This might then be followed by working through his low self-esteem, his feelings of not deserving more and his self-consciousness.

How we look to the external environment to help us with our troublesome emotions can result in anything from its avoidance or denial to its expression or discharge, thus determining our focus, what we see and don't see, in other words, our reality. Here are some examples of how various people assess their environment and thereby distort, or completely don't see, various aspects of reality:

- A person suffering from low self esteem would be limited by their hesitancy, fear of exposing themselves, and their reluctance to be definite.
- A person still troubled by a past characterized by severe deprivation would likely experience the world as cold, unrewarding, or rejecting and have little confidence or interest in understanding it.
- A person dominated by a strict conscience would fear criticism, become absorbed in how others might view their behavior, and find themselves less sensitive to the adaptive aspects of reality.
- A depressed person's inertia and withdrawal would severely limit their awareness of the world and their ability to process it.
- An anxious person's take on reality would be limited by their focus on how the environment might affect them.
- An angry person might be preoccupied with finding an object to criticize or punish.

- And, last but not least, a person lacking gratifying experiences in reality might be seeking love and looking for a suitable object upon which to project some profoundly positive feelings. In their case, connecting with the reality, especially the reality of that person probably would not be very important or, in some cases, completely unwanted.

We must see ourselves as we really are, be honest with ourselves, and acknowledge and come to grips with our emotional conflicts. By connecting with reality (our own and that of the rest of the world) we are put in touch with something that we can trust. Our ability to adapt is increased because we are able to accept first our own reality and second that of the external world.

Now that we understand the importance of staying in reality, let's look at "Emma" and "Sally" as examples, respectively, of the impact of unresolved emotional issues on external reality and the gentle reward of being able to accept reality in relationships.

Sally was recently diagnosed with terminal breast cancer with bone metastases which caused her exquisite pain and required both chemo and radiation therapy. Sally's sister Emma, who lives about 500 miles away and was aware of her painful condition, called to say that she would be visiting near Sally around the time of Sally's birthday, and would like to come to help her celebrate it. She made this offer in three separate calls and each time emphasized "celebrate." Sally is not only in profound pain but dealing with her new death sentence and hardly in a position to celebrate anything. Emma is known for her rudeness, her insensitivity, and her sarcasm.

In their next telephone conversation, Emma announced that she had been "Googling" Sally's type of cancer. She then said "Now, Sally, you must drink plenty of water for your kidneys." She repeated this sentence three or four times in an exaggerated fashion—even giggling. She seemed to get delight out of this because Sally, an M.D. herself, was fully aware of such health considerations and wasn't seeking the advice of an amateur. From Sally's point of view, Emma appeared to be immersed in the joy of teasing her.

In a subsequent phone call, Emma expressed her hope that Sally was "getting better." Of course, someone in Sally's condition could "feel better" some days but she was not going to ever "get better." Emma bragged that her important husband was off on a business trip and that she would join him later in Singapore. She then again told Sally to "get better" in a sarcastic, overly enthusiastic, cheerleader manner. At the end of this conversation, Sally noticed that she had no discernible emotional response. However, soon after, she found herself wanting to call Emma back to confront her about her teasing, sarcasm and provocativeness, to point out her grandiosity about her husband, and to note that Emma does nothing in the way of trying to be kind or helpful. But she hesitated and found herself intrigued, actually fascinated, by trying to understand where Emma was "coming from."

Her thoughts turned to the idea that Emma may be doing this because nothing else in her life is meaningful; this is just the real Emma: angry, insulting, teasing, sarcastic, provocative, and grandiose. "Catching her in her anger" and confronting her with it no longer seemed like something Sally wanted to do. *"My sister is already stuck in her anger, already penalized by it, a non-achiever who needs something positive from me"*, she thought. Sally, because of her personal integrity, could comfortably accept Emma exactly as she was and felt no need to react to her anger or to confront her with it.

Sally continued to think about Emma and decided that perhaps Emma had been able to risk bringing her real self, as hostile as it might be, directly into this relationship with Sally as much as with anyone without making her uncomfortable or driving her away, maybe more than she ever had dared with her parents. This would mean that Sally is getting Emma a better experience than she ever had with them. Here, Emma was achieving a new height in risking her very essence with another. She may have discovered that she was fully heard and understood, that she made nobody uncomfortable nor drove anybody away, that there was absolutely no damage done by hurting another's feelings, and that a new respect, level of appreciation, and connection with her sister was achieved. Sally, with her personal integrity, had succeeded in providing a comfortable connection that the real Emma, with all her hostility, could easily accept. Now, let's see what the benefits of Sally's relaxed approach to Emma's hostility might be.

In the next conversation Emma opened up as never before. She mentioned that she had not visited her children in over a year, that she felt that her husband's travels preempted her trips, that she was lonely and bored, and couldn't accomplish anything. Here, at last, there was little or no provocative behavior. She was openly, honestly, and spontaneously sharing with Sally her sorrows, which Sally listened to and calmly accepted. Emma showed no hostility or sarcasm about Sally's painful situation. It's clear that Emma finally felt heard and connected to, in spite of her previous expressions of hostility and attempts to drive Sally away. Sally realized Emma probably experiences her anger as rejection, that is, "*if I'm angry, I will be rejected.*" At this point, she was no longer attempting to push people away with her bristling sarcasm.

In a subsequent conversation Emma spoke intimately regarding her marriage, much more than ever before. She talked about how her relationship with her husband was very limited by his coming home late, drinking, and excusing himself to work on his computer. She said that she really provided little for him other than nice meals when he was in town. She concluded with "at least he hasn't kicked me out of the marriage!" At this point, Sally felt she had achieved a real, meaningful connection with Emma that was both very gratifying and satisfying to both of them. Sally's achieving a connection with Emma, the reality of it for better or worse, was an end in itself. Emma discovered that she was capable of sharing her true feelings with her sister and how safe and gratifying this could be. Heretofore, it was more than she had been willing to risk. Here, we could say that Emma grew emotionally.

In addition to helping us achieve personal integrity, connecting to reality is an end in itself. It allows us to see first ourselves, then others, and finally "the world" as we and they really are. This gives us trustworthy information to help us understand, accept, and cope with ourselves and the outer world. Knowing and accepting ourselves, our feelings, and our wishes gives us the greatest chance of viewing the rest of the world accurately. When we don't know or accept ourselves, our ability to assess ourselves is reduced, the boundaries between us and the world become blurred, and our perceptions of the world are distorted by the emotions we have projected onto the outer world. This means that we begin to respond to the outer world (reality) with perceptions that are inaccurate or irrelevant. This penalizes us with the world in general and people in particular. In addition and of course primarily, our unresolved troublesome feelings interfere with our personal joy, versatility and our just plain humanism.

Part 2: Anger

Frustration and anger are feelings we all have. This is a given. The crucial issue is how skillful we become at handling them. At its core, anger is a signal that our expectations of gratification of our wishes are out of sync with reality and in need of recalibration. Given this, anger offers a clue that there are aspects of reality that we have been unable to accept. Learning to understand anger helps us to develop personal integrity because whenever we begin to comprehend something in the world, we gain a better ability to cope with it and/or control it. Anger is no exception. Anger is a very real part of our human existence and must be understood for our adaptation and brought under our control because of its potential for destructive behavior.

Again, anger comes from our inability to accept the frustration of unmet wishes. From childhood on, we all will, at times, experience frustration. And anger is our natural reaction to frustration. The amount of anger a given person has is a function of the amount of frustration to which they are subjected and their ability to cope with the ensuing anger.

The most efficient way to reduce anger is to identify the source of frustration and recalibrate expectations to agree with what reality will actually provide. This is accomplished by the following sequence:

- First, we need to become aware of our anger. Some people are very skillful at recognizing it and others are not. In general, people who are able to identify and accept their anger tend to have less of it and those less able to do so tend to have more.
- Second, once we are aware of our anger we must search for its source. Invariably, there will be some wishes or expectations we have that the environment is not meeting. These frustrated wishes need to be identified.
- Third, once we have identified the wishes which the environment is not and will not gratify, we must then begin to emotionally accept the reality of this pending lack of gratification. Only then will our anger start to subside.

Once anger is understood, it can become completely innocuous and serve as a tremendous source of understanding, an absolutely priceless promoter of human growth and evolution. This means then that anger, per se, is not destructive. It is just a feeling in response to how we perceive the environment.

As you now understand, anger is always a signal that one of our expectations is being frustrated. A mature, evolved person can accept that the world didn't go the way they wanted it to: they were able to identify their disappointment, accept it, and make the best of things. This may subsequently involve grieving over a loss (dealing with the remaining wish). But so often, one gets angry, doesn't accept it, feels cheated, and maligns the world or somebody in it.

When you begin to understand the anger that you already have in your life, you will then have less of it. Any time we feel hurt or annoyed by another's criticism, it suggests that a part of us that is in agreement with them has been mobilized. Understanding this alerts us to one of our internal conflicts and now gives us a chance to come to grips with it.

In the verbal arena we can safely accept an unlimited amount of anger. Here we have a forum where it can become, via understanding, an asset for very human and meaningful interactions resulting in resolution of conflict, personality growth, evolvement, and even catharsis. With respect to catharsis, an angry person's unrest is often decreased by their heated verbal discharge to the point where they are much less in danger of acting out their rage physically. They may even begin to identify their own unreasonable expectations of the world. This is especially true if the listener is able to comfortably hear and accept what is said as meaningful and worthy of being understood.

Most of us do not understand the positive outcomes that anger can affect, therefore, it tends to be barred from interpersonal relationships. It causes most people to be uncomfortable and even to withdraw from a relationship. It causes many people to feel hurt and many to malign others. It causes some to respond with more anger either verbally or physically. In short, it tends to destroy relationships because its discharge is misunderstood and therefore destructive rather than constructive, even in the verbal arena.

Now that we understand the meaning of anger a little bit better, when we encounter an incensed person we can respond by considering what aspects of reality they are having trouble accepting rather than responding to their fury with our own emotions. Yet, unfortunately, so often, in the face of anger one emotionally withdraws and lapses into their previously acquired discomfort with it. This relapse has nothing to do with the current relationship or any aspect of the external reality. Moreover, this relapse into one's emotional conflict is often misidentified as part of the external reality (an aspect of the relationship). This reaction is not adaptive and means that neither person is coming to the encounter from a place of personal integrity.

Let's look at two examples of anger being handled constructively by personalities demonstrating integrity:

"Grandpa" is visiting his daughter's family over the Fourth of July. He's sort of a crotchety old man and goes to bed early, probably having already forgotten it's a holiday. It's not dark yet and the family is lingering on the patio drinking beer and having a good time. Grandpa's bedroom is close to the patio and his window is open on this warm summer night. He's opened and closed his window several times with a purposeful bang. Finally he appears on the patio and begins to give the family a hard time for making so much noise. He has their attention and they calmly listen. All of a sudden, a string of firecrackers goes off next door. He takes obvious note of this, appears to understand why, and seems to calm down a little. Then a cherry bomb goes off. At this point he throws up his hands, rolls his eyes, and pleasantly says, "Okay, have a good night" and saunters off to bed with a smile from everyone in the family.

In this simple example, Grandpa's wish to go to sleep was not being gratified. The source of his anger, the environment not accommodating his wish for sleep, is easily identified. Once he realizes that it will not be met due to the holiday, he accepts reality and his anger disappears!

"Jim" and "David" have been together for many years. When David finished stating his preference for what they might do that evening Jim replied, "Damn you! You're always trying to control everything. Why do we always have to do it your way? You never give me a chance... I was all ready to tell you what I wanted to do and you began. You never listen to me." He continued, "Sometimes I know what I want to do and other times I don't. This time I did but I didn't know how to put it without being too aggressive. So, I guess I was a little slow in stating what I wanted." David replied," You know, I did wait but you didn't say anything." Jim replied, "I always feel I have to be forceful with you whenever I announce my wishes but I worry I'll be offensive." Jim continued, "Now that I think of it, that's what held me back. As a child my wishes were always rejected, my parents made me feel selfish and rude for asking. Actually, now whenever I do get my way, I feel greedy!" David replied, "I am glad to see that you're risking feeling greedy!"

Here is a couple that is clearly comfortable with anger. Initially, Jim erroneously identified David as one of the characters from his past that had thwarted his wishes. He unwittingly projected his troublesome feelings on to David; unaware that the anger he felt was actually coming from his own unresolved issues. However, neither escalated the anger, instead, they identified the wishes that were not being met in the present reality and the unresolved conflict this moment stimulated. This allowed them to work out some of their personal problems in the relationship with each other.

Anger is a part of our humanness and one of our more important feelings. We need to learn to accept it so that it dissipates and is no longer available for discharge, either verbally or physically. In the verbal arena, anger is frequently the first indication of a problem in need of a solution and often the only way an individual can reveal it to themselves or the world.

Therefore, whenever anger appears, a premium must be placed upon it. As we have learned, first, we accept the other person's ire; we remain interested in it and invite them to talk about it. Then, we look for the source of it and we invite them to fully explore for what they blame us. This is accomplished by our profound comfort with, understanding and acceptance of, and interest in anger.

By regularly and routinely recognizing our anger and treating it as a signal that our wishes are not being gratified by reality and are thereby in need of recalibration, we can evolve ourselves emotionally. This will happen by identifying and resolving our conflicts stemming from unrealistic expectations of the world, unrealistic because reality just did not, is not, or will not gratify our wishes/expectations regardless of how legitimate, deserving or fair they may have seemed. If we approach anger as above, then these things follow:

1. All anger in the verbal arena can be accepted.
2. An angry, critical opinion never diminishes the recipient even if it is accurate–it just increases understanding.
3. At no time will an opinion ever warrant an apology.
4. Accepting anger by understanding it is much easier than avoiding it.

5. Anger is never irrational. It is rational with respect to one's unrealistic expectations; it is the expectations that are irrational.

While frustration and anger are a natural part of all of our lives, hopefully we aren't confronted with more than we can learn to handle.

Part 3: The Thrust to Grow or *In Statu Nascendi*

There is an obvious thrust to grow in all living things. For example, even when a young plant is stepped upon and flattened, if it survives it will continue to seek the sun albeit with a kink in its stem. In humans there is a thrust to grow both physically and mentally. With respect to the latter, this thrust is both emotional and intellectual and is an ever present aspect of living. I like to call it *in statu nascendi:* our natural thrust to evolve. Our innate thrust to evolve helps us somehow bust out of our restrictive stance and find a better means of reducing frustration, hurt or resentment. To do so may involve placing oneself in troublesome situations much like the ones in our childhood that we found overwhelming. By re-confronting the dragon, so to speak, we hope that somehow, this time, we can come out on top by evolving in ways that were not possible before. We have no idea *how* this might happen, we just feel that we must go back to where we were last emotionally overwhelmed. We attempt to set this up by provoking a similar situation with our anger and go from there, often without our awareness or conscious control. As we shall see in Chapter 3 where we discuss Active Understanding, this thrust can be facilitated by another's awareness and appreciation, and particularly by their comfort, with our situation, often without our even knowing it. This means that the presence of a person who is more comfortable with our emotional struggles will help us in our thrust to grow.

This thrust to evolve is strong in personalities with integrity, perhaps because risking has been reinforced by their previous success in doing so. However, their thrust to evolve may be more subtle and less evident because they do not need to rely so much on another's comfort level or, at least not as blatantly, as one with a personality that has not yet evolved does.

During my years of practice, the thrust to grow seemed especially prominent and occurred regardless of the patient's awareness, cooperativeness, honesty, or apparent "motivation for therapy." Let's look at some examples of this thrust to grow:

"Joanne" is a professional woman in her fifties with mild bouts of depression. After about six months of weekly psychotherapy, she reported that she was beginning to look forward to coming to my office and to experience joy during our meetings. She usually chose to stand in the waiting room and always had a smile on her face and a twinkle in her eye when I opened the door. One day she paused and with definite dread said "Oh, my God, I'm not supposed to be doing this!" with respect to her newfound happiness as she entered the office. Joanne had not expected this delight or her reaction to it. She had not even been aware of the absence of this kind of pleasure in her other relationships. Most of her life had been spent working hard at her profession and achieving a great deal of success. It seemed as though whatever enjoyment she had in life had been earned through hard work. Here, in psychotherapy, she experienced joy in a relationship just for its existence for the first time. Joanne's mother had classic schizophrenia and it was easy to hypothesize that she found no happiness in the relationship offered by her mother. Despite her sense of doing something forbidden, she continued attending our sessions until she was fairly comfortable in accepting her gladness, the very same feeling that had been unavailable to her in her early relationship with her mother. As her therapist, my understanding, appreciation, and especially my comfort with her daring to risk this forbidden joy of her childhood, facilitated Joanne's natural thrust to evolve. Hopefully, she has gone on to find that she can spontaneously experience and accept this new pleasure in her other relationships.

Let's look at another example. "Mary" was a single forty-five-year-old government employee who lived alone. She experienced occasional bouts of psychosis which generally lasted only a few days and were not accompanied by much disorganization. She rarely missed work. She was an accomplished artist but had never dared to exhibit her paintings. One day she found the nerve to hang one on her living room wall, reported that it was too self-aggrandizing, despite the fact that she lived alone and had had no recent visitors, and promptly regressed emotionally with a brief episode of craziness. As her therapist, all I could do was remain comfortable with her perceived self-aggrandizing audacity when she reported hanging her painting on her living room wall and, especially with her reporting that she did not back off and take the painting down. In short, she risked exposing her essence as never before, reacted with a brief episode of madness, and quickly recovered without backing off. I feel that this was a period of emotional growth for her and hope that she will keep risking and growing.

Now here's one more: "Ann" is a thirty-year-old, employed, single woman who had graduated from college Phi Beta Kappa. She also had a mother with chronic schizophrenia. She was planning a trip to Europe but felt very guilty about doing so. She worried she was being too selfish doing something so nice for herself. Warily, she revealed her plans to her mother, who lived about fifty miles away. Ann's mother responded by beginning to show signs of going crazy again. Ann announced that she had canceled her trip and her mother's symptoms disappeared. The relationship between Ann's thrusts for independence and pleasure and her mother's response of showing symptoms of schizophrenia was quite evident to Ann intellectually and we discussed it many times. With obvious trepidation, she reinstated her plans to go to Europe, whereupon her mother promptly became crazy enough to require hospitalization. Ann then felt so selfish for catering to her own pleasures that she canceled her trip once and for all. And, shortly thereafter, her mother was discharged from the hospital. Unfortunately, Ann could not sustain her thrust for independence, although I would like to think that intellectually she made some progress in this direction. Again, as her therapist, my appreciation and comfort level with her attempts at independence were the best that I could give her. It would not have been appropriate for me to have advised her to go or not to go to Europe. I don't know if she ever got there.

While I do not know how this turned out, let's look at the possibilities for both of them to grow. It would be my hope that Ann eventually became comfortable enough with her thrusts for independence that she could openly schedule a trip to Europe, calmly announce it to her mother, and take the trip with ease and enjoyment. It is further my hope that Ann would learn to execute her thrusts for independence so comfortably and convincingly that her mother would forgo future attempts to control her through episodes of craziness and hospitalizations. In short, Ann's acquiring comfort with and skill in exhibiting her independence would not only evolve her but eliminate the secondary gain in her mother's bouts of psychosis. Here, the mother would be invited to grow by accepting her daughter's independence, freedom, and capacity to enjoy because her attempts to control are no longer working. In this way both of them could obtain more personal integrity.

Part 4: Nature & Nurture

Scientific observation is entirely non-judgmental. According to scientists, the world and its contents are products of nature and nurture and therefore cannot be judged. As we shall see, human beings too, are products of their nature and nurture, and are, therefore unable to be judged. In fact, true understanding precludes judgments of all things, including people.

From this we can conclude that all creatures are just what one would expect given what they are born with and the subsequent conditioning they received from their environment. This also means that human beings are neither "good" nor "bad"; they are just doing what any human being would do with the particular genetic inheritance with which they entered the world and the world's subsequent effects on that over time.

However, so often we declare something or someone innately "good" or "bad" and when we do, we actually leave the external reality and enter a world of judgment entirely of our own creation. We become immersed in our feelings and leave the reality of the relationship. And our regression from reality doesn't stop there. We come to believe that *the other person* is the *cause* of our unrest instead of our own internal conflict.

And finally, in a third stage in our sequence of regression from reality, we declare them "bad" and further depart from the here-and-now of the relationship into the meaningless reality we have created.

This is not to say that the behavior of humans cannot be destructive or that their destructiveness need not be addressed by society, for example, incarceration for those who have committed crimes or pose a threat to others. It merely means that human beings are most often "doing their thing" which is neither good nor bad for their particular circumstances. Given this, a person's very being cannot be judged as either "good" or "bad". Furthermore, we will no longer say someone is a "bad" person, but rather we can estimate their potential for destructive behavior and need for rehabilitation. Likewise, we will no longer say that someone is a "good" person, but rather describe their potential for constructive behavior. If we make this distinction, namely, our *beings,* versus our deeds or behavior, we will be less inclined to leave reality and let our own internal conflicts interfere and, therefore, maintain our personal integrity.

Let's consider times when we do the opposite by declaring others as "good" people. This usually occurs because they make us feel good about ourselves—they meet some of our emotional needs such as flattering us, being generous with us, etc. Declaring them, their beings, as "good" has nothing to do with the present external reality. It is, again, a creation of ours that has nothing to do with external here and now in the same way as when we pronounce them as "bad." In both cases we are simply placing a value upon their being, something that is, as we have seen, not "judgeable".

Love and hate are also our reactions to a neutral world. They are values of our own creation, like good and bad but more intense, which we project upon the environment. Yet, so often, love and hate determine how we treat this neutral world regardless of its presenting reality. Our love and hate for objects or people are determined by *our emotional use of, or response to, these objects* or *people* and are not determined by *our understanding of them* or *of their way in the world.* This placing of love and hate upon the being of a person or an object is different from placing a value on its utility. For example: "John" wants to leave an island which, after a hurricane, is no longer connected by a bridge to the mainland. He has access to both a car and a boat. As far as his immediate needs, the boat is obviously of much more utility than the car. This determination is not a result of John's emotional reaction to the boat or the car such as "I love the boat and I hate the car," nor does it involve placing any intrinsic value upon either one, such as "good" boat or "bad" car. In this simple example, John reacts with personal integrity, the result of his realistic understanding approach.

With respect to the emotional states that interfere with objective observation and understanding, we have seen the importance of identifying our anger. When we are angry, as we have seen, it is a signal that our expectations are not being met. Until we recalibrate our expectations to be in sync with reality, we may feel as if the world is mistreating us and place a negative value - or judgment - upon it or some object or person. At this point we may become absorbed in our feelings of injustice or deprivation, which are derived from our past experiences. These feelings have nothing to do with the reality at hand and greatly compromise, if not preclude, our ability to perceive and understand reality without judgment. At times we may even malign objects in the world and try to effect harsh treatment. It is important to recall that all objects and people are simply products of their nature and nurture and are not the cause of our unrest. Judging them has absolutely nothing to do with reality.

Part 5: Narcissism

One of the greatest barriers to becoming a personality with integrity is the tendency to narcissistic behavior. In order to live fully with integrity, it is important to understand narcissism and how it functions, often without our realizing it, in everyday encounters.

Narcissism is defined by Webster's Dictionary as:

1. Self love; excessive interest in one's own appearance, comfort, importance, abilities, etc.;
2. In psychoanalysis, arrest at, or regression to, the first stage of sexual development in which the self is an object of sexual pleasure.

For our purposes, we will use the first definition and add to it "one's own interpretation of the world."

The narcissist's focus and interpretation of the world tends to be based on their feelings. The more narcissistic a person is, the more they feel entitled to judge others and to discharge their feelings upon the world. We now understand that the world and its contents are simply products of nature and nurture, therefore judgment as to their inherent goodness or badness is entirely unwarranted. Narcissists, however, are unable to get past their emotional needs in order to objectively perceive and treat the world. They interpret the world according to their feelings as well as their needs. Further, they tend to expect the world to cater to those needs in order to sustain them emotionally. At times of difficulty, they often malign certain objects and recommend punishment. This maligning may allow them to justify the discharge of their angry feelings upon the world and provide an illusion of their control over it.

We all produce love and hate according to our needs and associate one or the other with an object or person in the outer world. However, a narcissistic person doesn't stop here. A narcissistic person will project these feelings of love or hate upon the environment and then use these projections to justify their behavior.

Let's look at a few examples. "Laura" is in the terminal stages of pancreatic cancer and experiencing constant pain. Her son "Michael" feels better when he can make his mother feel better, that is to say he is primarily motivated by his own needs. He visits his mother, hugs and strokes her, then looks at her in a pleading way, and asks, "You feel better now, don't you?" When Laura doesn't answer that she does, Michael may become angry because his primary wish to make *himself* feel better by helping his mother is not gratified.

In a similar manner, Michael often stocks his mother's kitchen with expensive foods that go uneaten because Laura has no appetite for those particular kinds of foods. This further annoys Michael because, again, his goal is to satisfy his need to make himself feel better by experiencing himself as the cause of her feeling better—as opposed to a primary wish to attempt to meet her therapeutic needs.

In contrast, his older sister "Eileen" visits Laura with the primary motivation to meet her mother's appropriate needs regardless of whether or not she receives her mother's praise. She understands and comfortably accepts when she can't make her mother feel physically better. In a similar manner, she actively discerns what foods their mother needs and can eat, she then provides those and comfortably accepts whatever Laura can or cannot eat. Eileen is not helping to make herself feel better. In other words, she is not acting from a place of narcissism.

More poignantly, when it comes time for consideration of Laura to go to a hospice to die, Eileen would make the decision solely on the basis of Laura's needs whereas Michael, the more narcissistic personality, would likely make the decision based on his needs. He might say something like "Mom, *I couldn't stand* to see you suffer, so I sent you to the hospice," thereby putting his own narcissistic need to feel better before his mother's best interest.

Here's another example of how narcissism can play out. There is a beggar by a stop sign on the side of the road. Many drivers are happy to pause and hand him cash without any knowledge of what might really be best for him, as they are primarily motivated by their own wish to give and, therefore, feel good about themselves. Passively acquired money may not always be the best thing for him. It is possible that the most helpful thing for the beggar would be for somebody to consider first what's best for the beggar and say to him, "You look like the kind of guy who could hold down a job" and the beggar might reply, "You know, with your confidence, I'm gonna try." He may then go out and find a job thanks to one driver's resisting the narcissistic urge to feel good about himself by handing money out the window. It should be acknowledged that it is entirely possible for a driver motivated by a wish to do what's best for the beggar to give money without any knowledge of his true needs simply because the driver accepts operating on the probability that he needs money.

Here's another example with the same beggar and a different driver. This driver, "Claire," is a little more grandiose and self-serving. There are a number of people in her car whom she wants to impress. She ostentatiously hands the beggar a $20 bill which he takes with great deliberateness and a big contrived smile. When Claire drives off, he then gives her the finger with great exaggeration. He understood that her generosity was purely to gratify her need to look good in front of her friends and that she was using him as a vehicle for this narcissistic gratification. Let's go a bit further into his actions. Her treatment angered him, and, as we now know, anger is a signal of the mobilization of an unresolved emotional conflict. We could guess that the beggar is, understandably, uncomfortable with the feelings of humiliation associated with his situation which were mobilized by Claire's use of him for her own grandiosity. He became immersed in these feelings and left the external reality with his angry reaction. Here, both parties lost their personal integrity: she by using the environment (the beggar) to support her self-esteem, and he by discharging his anger upon her instead of accepting it for understanding. Had Claire's primary motivation been to do what was best for him, he probably would have realized it by her sincerity and graciously accepted her money.

When we begin to use the world primarily for the gratification of our immediate personal emotional needs we lapse into narcissism. The signal for this is our love or hate. We begin to look for objects in the real world upon which to express our love or hate. *Narcissism is the expression or discharge of these feelings upon neutral objects in the world.* At this point, all personal integrity has been lost. I like to think of the narcissistic default as a coin with two sides: one of love and one of anger.

Let's take a further look at how love and hate play out in narcissism. Any expression of love or hate is an action that arises entirely within us in our response to a neutral world. As such, it is entirely narcissistic. Here are a few examples:

- *"I am angry and I want to hurt somebody to make myself feel better even if discharging these feelings is detrimental to others or to society."* The narcissism here is quite evident when we recall that the world and its objects are products of their nature and nurture and are, therefore, neutral, not warranting destructive treatment. Yet, here the narcissist is saying *"I want to use these objects solely for my needs."* This is a long way from acceptance of the world based upon understanding. Furthermore, even if this discharge of anger occurred upon the enemy during a war, it might very well have been contrary to our wisest and best military tactics, for example, killing an enemy soldier who might be a valuable source of information. It is based entirely on irrationality.

- *"I want to love, I need an object to love."* Here, the narcissist's view is that the function of the object is to meet his/her own personal needs to love something. He might want to worship them, fuss over them, cater to their needs as he has determined them, possess them, protect them, control them, etc. These very likely would have nothing to do whatsoever with what might be best for that person, the love object. There is no evidence here of a personality with integrity which might best determine the reality or needs of the other person and lead to some mutuality. One can see that the narcissist would quickly become disappointed in this relationship if the other had enough positive self-esteem to not need worshiping, the wherewithal not to need to be taken care of, protected, or possessed, etc. Moreover, someone with these needs, in this case wanting to express pure love, would be disappointed if they got to know the real person because reality would intrude upon their preferred narcissistic perception. Often a pure love relationship is an attempt to avoid the reality of that person or the reality of a relationship. And, not surprisingly, as the reality breaks through, these types of relationships end. Most of us can vouch for this!

- The golfer who attempts to use his game to support his self-esteem. No matter how well he plays it's never good enough and most of the time he is angry and complaining. His dependency upon the environment to enhance his self-esteem interferes with the joy and meaningfulness available to him from the reality of just playing the game.

Put simply, narcissism interferes with personal integrity because it is characterized by a limited ability to get beyond one's own emotional needs. A narcissistic default results in a compromised ability to perceive, understand, and deal effectively with reality.

Now that we have looked at various aspects of our personality that contribute to or interfere with our personal integrity, it's time to learn how to achieve it.

Chapter 3:

———◆◆◆———

Active Understanding

Part 1: Why is active understanding important?

The *active understanding approach* to our inner thoughts and feelings is important because it gives us our best chance to "get beyond ourselves." When we can do this we experience a level of comfort with ourselves and can turn to the outer world without seeking to gratify our emotional needs there which can interfere with our perception of reality. On the contrary, when we are unable to comfortably accept and understand our own thoughts and feelings we are troubled and look to our external environment for help. Seeking help from the external environment to sustain ourselves emotionally compromises our ability to perceive and to understand the world around us. Active understanding and accepting our thoughts and feelings allows us to avoid the narcissistic defaults which seek gratification in the outer world and interfere with its perception and understanding

Active understanding leads to an accurate assessment of reality, and active understanding of anger allows one to identify how reality is not accommodating his or her expectations. Once identified, one can bring their expectations of gratification of their wishes into accord with reality. When this happens anger subsides. This is adaptive behavior and indicates that the personality has maintained its integrity.

Active understanding increases our awareness of reality and, therefore, our subsequent ability to deal with that reality. This is true not only in the world in general but in human relationships in particular. The maintenance of an understanding approach further protects us from withdrawing into our own internal problems, casting judgment, and/or discharging some of our feelings which are inappropriate to the immediate environmental situation.

Let's take a look at some of the advantages of active understanding in an interpersonal situation. In a relationship with an angry person, understanding makes it possible to appreciate their troubled circumstances without responding personally to their anger. This can be true even when they direct it at us. They are the one with the problem, that is, they have the anger, and we can benefit them with our understanding without introducing an unrelated problem of our own even though they may prefer to see it this way, i.e., that we are the ones with the anger. The more we understand about them, their circumstances, what problems or conflicts with which they are struggling, where they are coming from: their fears, their ambitions, their misconceptions, their furtive attempts at self-assertion, what self-critical parts of themselves they project upon us, etc., the better we are able to help them in resolving their problem. Our comfortableness with their risk, generated by our active understanding, is probably the most helpful thing. All of this creates trust and confidence in a safe ongoing relationship, just the supportive/facilitative environment that they need. We get to know them in much more depth and our interest in and appreciation of them can only grow. This provides for solid, in depth, meaningful, interesting ongoing relationships. *I like to think that the greatest gift one person can give another is being comfortable with them and accepting them based on understanding. Or especially to be more comfortable with them with their feelings and with their attempts to grow then they are.* This is especially true when the other person is having trouble accepting their self and/or their feelings and we are more comfortable with them than they are with themselves.

With active understanding there is no opinion that will ever require an apology. This is a very profound statement, but, I think, absolutely true. Just think about it! This is because the listener remains in the understanding mode and does not take anything personally, therefore, no one is hurt and understanding is increased. Freedom of speech doesn't mean that we will always risk presenting our true feelings. However, if we can expect to be understood, the probability is high that we will risk speaking our true feelings and actually have more freedom of speech, another profound idea! The mere decreeing of freedom of speech does little to increase it compared to the expectation that what is said will be understood, comfortably accepted, genuinely appreciated, and lead to facilitative solutions. When active understanding becomes effective in a relationship, confidence in the relationship grows to the point that the participants may risk any and all aspects of themselves. In short, *"If you can think it, say it. We'll deal with it."* That would be true freedom of speech; anything less is a compromise, and, compromises in interpersonal relationships threaten personal integrity.

Part 2: How does active understanding work?

The first step in active understanding is to listen to what the other person has to say and regard the complaint as their legitimate and best perception or degree of understanding. Even if they are angry at us and their criticism is accurate, it doesn't mean that our being is flawed, since, as we know, we too, are products of our nature and nurture. Their criticism first must be accepted as their current perception or understanding, not something to be taken personally. Our goal is to try to understand their predicament, their struggle, their confusion, how they may be hurting and what they may be risking in an effort to come to grips with something or to grow emotionally. Even if their criticism is accurate, we still want to understand why they are so angry with the reality of our unacceptable behavior. Hopefully, we can accept their criticism of us with interest and appreciation. Often the mere verbalization of their perceived deprivation and our acceptance of it as a concern warranting understanding calms them down, and may even result in their more accurate assessment of their own wishes and reality.

Second, we must listen with a sense that the alleged source of anger needs to be examined. We hear their concerns with interest, respect, and a sense of legitimacy and calm so that they begin to experience us more as an assistant in unraveling their own conflicts and less as an adversary who is the cause of their anger. Their wish now has the best chance to be understood and the probability of the environment gratifying it determined. If it is impossible or improbable that the world can gratify their wish, then they can start to renounce their wish. At a time when they are angry and correctly blame us for their problem, we can not only correct the issue but try to understand why they are so angry at us.

Let's take a look at different outcomes of an encounter. First, we will examine what happens when one person does not use active understanding and then the same situation when they maintain their personal integrity through active understanding. Imagine we have a friend whom we see occasionally at social gatherings. They have a reputation for being inordinately passive at times and overly aggressive at others. During their aggressive moments they are given to being outrageous, shocking others, or embarrassing them, for example, "your slip is showing" or "there is a booger in your nose." They themselves do not appear to be comfortable with either of their techniques and seem to be struggling. In our conversation with them at this particular gathering they remark with unprovoked hostility that we have ugly blue eyes. (While this may seem like a simplistic example, perhaps too uninteresting to become excited about, I wanted an encounter in which you would not become emotionally absorbed and would be quickly able to resume your logical thinking.) This could be handled in several different ways. Let's look at this from our point of view first and then from their point of view.

From our point of view, let's take the worst case scenario first, where we do not employ active understanding and therefore, lose our personal integrity. We "take this personally," we begin to feel uncomfortable, even perhaps emotionally hurt, start to withdraw, to blame them as the source of our discomfort, to label them as "bad," and to want to punish them. Now, needless to say, this is a common response. What we need to recognize is that this response suggests that we ourselves have some difficulty accepting our eyes just the way they are; otherwise such a comment would not have bothered us. It is also possible that we are uncomfortable with the anger implied by their adversarial stance due to our own unresolved issues around the expression of anger.

Many of us would simply withdraw ourselves entirely from the relationship and the connection with the other person would be lost. We then, in all probability, would identify the other person as the source of our hurt, completely overlooking our own discomfort or conflict with our own blue eyes and/or with anger. And finally, we might malign the other person–pronounce them "bad" and consider revenge.

As you can see, taking this remark personally has resulted in emotional withdrawal from the external here-and-now reality and regression into our hurt stemming from our own internal conflict. If we believe that the other person is the primary source of our unrest, we have, in the strongest terms, a delusion. Our maligning another person's being as "bad" has no meaning in reality since human beings are products of their nature and nurture and therefore neither good nor bad. We have left the external reality; have lost our working connection with the other person, as well as our personal integrity. This is a terrible price to pay for our own failure to try to actively understand what the other person is about, perhaps merely trying to get our attention, and our regressing into our own unrelated emotional problems which suggests a personality with little or no integrity.

In this example, someone tries to make contact with us by telling us that we have ugly blue eyes (external reality) and we respond by emotionally reliving our long-standing discomfort with our blue eyes learned in our childhood (internal reality) that has nothing to do with the external reality. When we look at it this way, how could our response be any more inappropriate?

Now, again from our point of view, the best scenario is one in which we are absolutely comfortable with their anger and maintain a calm, comfortable, inquisitive, inviting focus upon them; in other words, we engage in active understanding and maintain our personal integrity. We are very interested in the real source of their angry "blue eyes" remark and why it is surfacing in their greeting of us at this time. We are pretty sure that we are not the real source of their anger, but we are comfortable with hearing from them about the possibility of being its true and legitimate source. We do not expect them to be able to explain the cause of their anger, although they may know or, in all probability, think that they know what it is. But we are able to discern that they are clearly in their aggressive mode as opposed to their passive mode. At this point we can't say much about the cause of their abrasiveness but find ourselves wondering about how they were brought up and where they are coming from now.

Simply by our staying in the *active understanding mode* and without knowing much about what's driving them, we notice that they now feel that they have our attention. They begin to talk comfortably with us about some recent interesting event in their life which we enjoy hearing. Unlike some of the other people in the room who were offended and wandered off, we maintain the connection with them, which we hope will become ongoing and provide us with more interesting stories. We also avoid any judgment of their being and thus remain in the current reality. Hopefully, they will have discovered that rough talk is not necessary for getting our attention and our relationship with them now will be a little deeper, more meaningful, confident, and trusting. We have maintained our personal integrity by seeking to actively understand their anger rather than taking it personally.

Now let's examine it from their position; first, the negative side, when we do not respond with active understanding. Their attempt to establish contact with us, namely, "you have ugly blue eyes," was met by our emotional discomfort and withdrawal. They feel discouraged that the abrasiveness of their best active attempt to assert themselves was not only obviously uncomfortable for them, but resulted in our being turned off, their being rejected and a distancing, or even suspension, of the relationship. They now regress to their passive mode, disappointed by their failure to connect with us. In all probability, their self-esteem remains low.

On the other hand, when we seek to actively understand their remark, that is we meet their "you have ugly blue eyes" with comfortableness and sympathetic attention, they discover that their abrasiveness was not necessary in order to get our attention. They know this because we did not respond with any intimidation or anger of our own and yet they still got our undivided attention. Given this experience, we might expect that their future attempts to get our attention will be less abrasive.

It is likely that they themselves are uncomfortable with their harsh approach and welcome the discovery of an effective alternative. This could signal the beginning of the resolution of their lifelong emotional conflict stemming from growing up in a home where one could only gain attention through some sort of rough assertion. It could be that they are having a better experience with us than they ever had with their parents! This experience with us will tend to endow our relationship with enduring trust and mutuality. And, of course, they had the pleasure of further connecting with us by sharing their stories. Here, because of our comfort based on understanding, we made a transition for them possible.

Obviously, our active understanding and calm in the face of the other person's anger tends to make the encounter with them much more benign. We outwardly accept the possibility of their angry projections upon us as true, but we never confirm them by reacting with anger. Failing to react with anger or hurt is a very powerful mediator, along with our calmness and comfort with their entire situation.

It should be clarified that accepting all of an individual's thoughts, feelings, or wishes as legitimate and worthy of consideration has nothing to do with permission to gratify, discharge, or act out a particular wish. For example, you might say: "Okay, so you want to rob a bank. I can accept the fact that you have this totally asocial impulse. Let's talk about your desire to rob a bank in the hopes that we can understand it, where it comes from, why it comes up at this time, etc." This reply in no way gives permission to rob a bank–in fact, understanding what robbing a bank will solve will probably lessen the thrust to do so. The same is true for the "ugly blue eyes" comment. In this case, our comfort with their provocative/hostile comment renders it harmless and absolutely denies them the sadistic gratification of any existing wish to hurt us.

The above example demonstrates that understanding of one individual by another can be practiced anytime, anywhere, and without their permission, cooperation, or knowledge. Moreover, a person exuding active understanding and ease with others is never intrusive – it is merely a comfortable acceptance of the other, their feelings, and their verbal expression and renders their hostility harmless.

What the process of active understanding suggests is that one person extend to another the same non-judgmental understanding (scientific observation) that we give to objects in the physical world which we routinely accept by their nature and nurture. *In essence, we are extending scientific observation to people without letting our feelings interfere just as we do with non-human objects.*

When we show genuine appreciation for an angry person's plight through practicing active understanding, we tend to calm them and not appear as their adversary. All this lessens the probability of a destructive outcome in the relationship.

Here is another example. At a book club where members eventually got to know each other very well, "Stacy", a young member well known for her crassness said to "Elaine", an older member "I hate you because you remind me of my mother." While this was clearly said to be provocative, there was also a tender, perhaps trusting element to it. Nevertheless, Elaine took offense and responded sarcastically, "Your mother must have been a wonderful woman," then walked off, and said, beyond Stacy's earshot, "She is malignant...I had a sister like her. If she stays around I'll just leave. The only thing I can think of is to stay out of her way...she should be jailed!" Elaine's angry response was common enough and worth examining.

Elaine, who always knew all about the authors, their previous books and myriad details of literature, could always substantiate whatever she said. She reacted with immediate anger and hurt feelings to Stacy's statement, albeit a little brusque and dramatic, by countering it and walking off, thus ending the connection. At this point Elaine is immersed in her own anger and has completely left the here-and-now reality of what Stacy might have really meant. She then judges Stacy to be bad, "malignant", and recommends punishment, that she be "jailed." She finds her so offensive that she threatens to leave the club just to avoid her. Given her remark about her sister, she is obviously subsumed by unresolved painful feelings stemming from her childhood, which are taking her completely out of the current reality. In all probability, Elaine identifies Stacy as the immediate cause of her unrest as opposed to Stacy's comment causing the mobilization of her own unresolved angry feelings which she still harbors toward her sister. In the strongest terms, this is a delusion. Elaine has taken herself out of the interpersonal reality and she is now at the mercy of her unresolved feelings. This is quite a price to pay and is not adaptive for either woman.

Now let's see where a little understanding might have taken them. In all probability this was, in part, Stacy's attempt to be provocative in a hostile sort of way, to be mean for the sake of hurting someone. In order for this to be meaningful for Stacy, the anger must be real, i.e., as in really trying to hurt somebody. At the same time, however, there was not only the acknowledgment of her anger, but a suggestion that she was willing to take the risk of trusting Elaine with some of her most troublesome feelings about her own mother. We might speculate that Stacy was willing to place more trust in Elaine than she ever was able to place in her own mother! Moreover, this may have been Stacy's bravest and best attempt to finally begin to get comfortable with her issues about her mother. In order for this to be meaningful, Stacy must risk involvement with her *real* anger that she is not yet in control of in a *real* relationship with another person. We can look at this as Stacy's attempt to get more comfortable with a disturbing feeling, namely her anger at her mother. She has always had trouble accepting her own anger and we can be sure of this because of her reputation for being crass, rude, and unkind; discharging her anger upon others in order to get rid of it (as opposed to accepting it so that it would not be available for discharge). Stacy expresses anger with an insightful comment about it. She appears to want to understand it–it being her *real* anger. This time she hopes that whatever hurt occurs will not be overwhelming to either party. And, at this point she has no idea about the acceptance of anger or how that might help her.

If Elaine could comfortably accept Stacy's anger, it would no longer be dangerous, no harm would have occurred, and Stacy could begin mastering it with her newfound comfort with it by borrowing on Elaine's comfort with it and the fact that her anger wasn't harmful or even disruptive.

This could have happened if Elaine had been entirely at ease with anger and not taken offense at Stacy's comment. Unfortunately, this did not happen; the feeling continued to be destructive now as it was in childhood with her sister. Thus Stacy was denied a chance to have been helped. It is important to understand that Stacy's attempt to get more comfortable with her anger *involved experimenting with her own sadism,* namely attempting to hurt Elaine for her own needs. This is necessary in order for the experience to be real enough to be meaningful.

Hence, as we speculated initially, this was an attempt on Stacy's part to use her anger in a mean way against Elaine. And, at the same time, it was a plea for help; her personal attempt to resolve her long-standing conflict with anger, that is, *"I have anger, I am unable to control it, and, therefore, I tend to discharge anger upon others."* If Stacy were able to be more explicit, she would continue by saying "I have done this since my childhood in relationships with others. This is my problem and the only way I know how to serve it up is to bring it into our relationship. *Help me find a different outcome. I have no idea how to resolve this other than to re-create it and hope for a better outcome."* It was also an opportunity for Stacy to help Elaine. Not so obviously, it was a chance for Elaine to build or consolidate her personal integrity. Let's take a look at this possibility.

Using active understanding, Elaine might have replied, "I thought maybe you hated me but I didn't know why. How do I remind you of your mother?" Stacy might have replied, "My mother was very accomplished, just like you, and she made me feel bad because I couldn't achieve her standards. When I see your efficiency, the whole issue comes up again and I feel bad." Elaine might have gone on to ask, "In what way do you see yourself as inefficient?" to which Stacy might have replied, "Everything I do... I feel bad about being so inept and when I see you, I feel even worse... even though you don't get mad at me, I still feel bad. How can you put up with my inefficiency?"

The conversation might continue like this:

Elaine: "Well, I feel I'm too efficient and too organized, to the point that I am not as spontaneous as I would like to be. Frankly, at times, I wish I had some of your disorganization so I could be a little freer and enjoy myself more."

Stacy: "But how can you put up with my inefficiency?"

Elaine: "Well, I admit that you are disorganized, in fact, at times terribly so."

After a silence, Stacy could reply, "You know, maybe I could try to be more organized and, now that I think of it, being sloppy seems to be a way of getting back at my mother." And, after a while she might add, "Gee, thanks. You've made me feel a lot better!"

I'd like to think that moving forward Stacy would be just a little bit more accepting, comfortable with, and in control of her anger than before. Even if she didn't resolve much emotionally, she might have gained some very valuable intellectual insight into her situation. She may also have acquired some optimism about approaching her anger. We can easily believe that the two women's relationship has gained a new awareness, a real mutual trust, and an appreciation of the other. Here, in this last version, Elaine further consolidated her personal integrity and avoided lapsing into judgment having little or nothing to do with reality or understanding.

When we accept the possibility of the other person's projections (hostile accusations) as true or accurate and yet fail to react with any discomfort or anger, their projections become something for them to understand. Actually and, parenthetically, their projections are true in the sense that they have an existence in reality, the reality being within themselves even though inaccurate with respect to the external world. It is like you are saying, *"Blaming me for your problems, even if it were true, is something I can comfortably accept and am able and ready to talk about."* We don't ever confirm their projections by reacting with irritation or by verbally agreeing, we just don't deny them. We allow them to exist as a possibility which we can accept for understanding. This gives the other person a new comfort with their accusations, distortions, or projections upon us, which then paves the way for them to accept them as their own, something originating within them. If they now can "own" their projection, they can begin to process it. Moreover, our comfort with their anger is now something upon which they can borrow from us. By borrowing upon our comfort and acceptance of their troublesome feelings, they can move toward understanding, accepting, and resolving conflict. The better we understand them, the more appropriate and effective we can be. Here, our own maturity, personal integrity and skills are being measured.

Here's a simple example. A person feels guilty about something they have done. They keep it to themselves, continue to feel miserable about it, and cannot deal rationally or effectively with it. Then, for whatever reason, they share their story with another person who listens and comfortably accepts it as regrettable but understandable. The perpetrator absorbs some of the other's comfort and now can re-approach their own misdeed with the options of appropriate acknowledgment, restitution, etc. All this occurs without any attempt to lessen or lower existing standards, to diminish the significance or destructive potential of the act, to demean the offended or the penalized or to even suggest forgiveness. In fact, nothing may have been said at all, just an obvious comfortable understanding and acceptance of their offensive behavior, allowing them to now comfortably and appropriately deal with it themselves.

While the process of active understanding may seem like we are devoting a lot of ourselves to help another person evolve, remember that we are the primary beneficiaries because we are maintaining our personal integrity and staying in reality. In the following example one partner maintains his personal integrity through active understanding, which allows the other partner to evolve. "John" is remarried to "Katie", a pretty, younger woman who had worked her way up to running the parks department of a rather large city. She came from a family that was so poor they swept up rice after weddings in order to get enough to eat. She could recall having been thrown out on the street because her mother couldn't pay the rent. Her father drank, was mean and physically abused her entire family. Vulnerability, anger, hurt, homelessness, fear, and hunger comprised her early memories. She had left home at the age of sixteen and made her way on her own from there. By forty she had raised a child, was divorced, and had to support only herself. She had no hobbies other than looking nice and cooking.

John had a small business that Katie could administrate. Because of her nice looks and cooking skills she was easily accepted into his group of friends. Over the next ten years she became extremely popular serving hors d'oeuvres which she might work on for the entire week. People could stand around with a glass of wine and eat her hors d'oeuvres for hours. Then she began to change. She stopped keeping a meticulous house. At times she was deliberately uncooperative and provocative with John. She became hostile. Their guests would come over as before, but her cooking had deteriorated. At times the house would not be tidy when the guests arrived. Moreover, at times she would do little or nothing in preparation for them. Some of her kindest guests would arrive early to do her cooking. Her big afternoons of magnificent hors d'oeuvres had diminished and she was left with only a few of her very best friends.

John understood that he had married a woman too eager to please and to meet his needs and to avoid her own. He seemed aware that she had, at least in the past ten years, avoided her troubled past by pleasing others. He sensed that now she was revisiting her angry, turbulent, disturbing history and could only hope that she'd fare better this time than she had in her childhood. Maybe this time her anger/rejection wouldn't be quite so painful; maybe the blame and self-recriminations wouldn't so effectively scar her self-image. Maybe her personal needs would emerge with some sense of legitimacy. And, maybe, this time she might find some parts of herself to enjoy.

John could appreciate that the risk Katie was taking required that she return to the real hostility, fear, and ugliness of her childhood environment. This was necessary so that she could start with her basic primitive un-evolved self and go from there, hoping to somehow come out better this time. The hope is that by re-exposing herself to the trauma, this time she will master the situation. Realistically, mastery of her situation will require many many revisits.

John's sense of understanding and failure to take offense helped facilitate this process. He was of the opinion that he could only get a better wife out of this and was happy to do whatever he could to help her as he had unwittingly exploited her emotional defenses earlier in the marriage. Slowly things began to change. He noticed that whereas before if he merely stated his position during a discussion, she would become angry, clam up, and withdraw for a few days, now, she would state her own opinion with some difficulty and be quite surprised to discover that her husband actually heard and honored her opinion. She didn't seem to quite know how to handle this and frequently felt herself rejected and her wishes held in contempt, contrary to John's comfortable acceptance of her position. At times John would return to the discussion days later in the hopes of fostering her acceptance of the legitimacy of her needs.

By initiating discussions in which he deliberately asked her to elucidate her thoughts, ideas, and wishes she could then pursue the positive emergence of her being without having to initiate hostile encounters. The encounters still got hostile at times, but only in reaction to her difficulties in accepting herself. At times she would get angry after John stated his preferences because she would misidentify this as something to which she was supposed to submit rather than something he simply wished her to hear.

After five years of this, Katie began to develop a positive sense of self. She could put her opinion out there, take joy in some other hobbies, and truthfully accept others' positions without feeling intruded upon. Her home became clean and tidy again and her cooking regained its former superiority, although it was now as a function of her wishes and her enjoyment of the process, not from a compulsion to please others. Her friends returned. Her husband's understanding, appreciation, and help with her thrust to grow made it easier for her and less burdensome for those around. Their relationship became, needless to say, deeper and more meaningful.

Part 3: Using active understanding on ourselves

If we practice active understanding with others, we may also practice it on ourselves. When we are alone and troubled or angry, we could allow a verbal outburst, then calmly stand back and review our cross words, then elucidate what aspect of reality we cannot accept, and then, finally, come to grips with our unrealistic expectations. Initially, this could be practiced in the shower while we are building confidence. In this way we can make anger work for us.

To see how self-analysis using active understanding might work, let's use the "you have ugly blue eyes" example again, this time in a situation where someone said it to me and I took it personally. I left the reality of the encounter by regressing deeply into my troubled feelings about my appearance.

In order to use active understanding on myself, I revisit the encounter in my spare time. First, I think back about what exactly was said that annoyed me. I begin to reflect on that, searching where my feelings of annoyance, hurt, or anger are the greatest. *I let myself become as immersed in my feelings as possible.* Surprisingly, I find my annoyance is not so much with what the person said, but with their adversarial stance. As I stay with my feelings, an image of my older brother comes up. I now begin to recall how uncomfortable I was with his competitiveness, specifically his adversarial stance, and, more specifically, the uncertainty about that because he was so much bigger than I physically. Here, I see my reaction had nothing to do with my blue eyes but merely the fact that my friend appeared to be assuming an adversarial position with me, and the indefiniteness of this in itself made me uncomfortable.

Now I would go further to let myself feel what it is about others being in an adversarial stance toward me that makes me so uncomfortable. I allow myself to experience the most intense aspects of my discomfort and eagerly watch for the images that might come to mind. The first image I sense was the uncertainty and fear on my brother's face once when we were out on the lake during a sudden storm and the waves got high. There were just the two of us; he was rowing against the wind and the waves, and I was sitting in the back of the boat looking directly into his face. I could swim, but not in those waves. At times I couldn't even see the shore. I was terrified and could do nothing. I turned to my brother for reassurance and all I could see was the uncertainty on his face. This lack of reassurance, the uncertainty of it, was terrifying.

Over the next few weeks I revisited this childhood trauma many times with my now adult mind and discovered that my uncomfortable reaction to it softened. As this happened, my older brother's smile began to appear. He had a small mouth with flat lips so that when he smiled it was sort of a grimace. But that wasn't it. I continued to reflect on his smile. Then it occurred to me that he would tease me by giving me that sadistic grin as he was about to bully me. Now that I think about it, that expression became enough to upset me and he rarely needed to bully me physically. I'm sure he liked to do this because he could get away with it in front of our parents. Amazingly, I had never thought about it before so clearly. No wonder I have been so ill-at-ease with uncertainty. Hopefully, my discomfort with ambiguity about an adversary's position will now lessen.

Other times, when I revisit my distress and annoyance with the "ugly blue eyes" comment, I re-experience anger with my mother. Early in my childhood, she often told me that I had "beautiful blue eyes." Somehow I now sense that I wanted her to say something more meaningful, more manly, something that reflected that she knew and felt what was going on inside me. "Beautiful blue eyes" seemed so empty and I wanted to feel a meaningful connection with her. I'm not sure I ever did. Later I decided that she was really reminding me that I had gotten *her* blue eyes. Given her apparent failure to have discerned what was really going on inside of me and her repeated reference to beautiful blue eyes, which she obviously had, I began to think about what a narcissist my mother must have been. No wonder I was so angry!

As I revisited my mother's comments I recalled that when I was a young teenager, her saying that I had beautiful blue eyes embarrassed me. At that time, like most adolescents, I was already self-conscious enough. Moreover, my masculinity wasn't well established then and I didn't find "little girl" compliments flattering. By discovering and emotionally revisiting these newly mobilized unresolved childhood conflicts, I find that my intolerance for uncertainty and ambiguity in interpersonal relationships has diminished.

Moreover, I am ultimately thankful for the "blue eyes" encounter as it led to the identification and resolution of restrictive elements of my personality. Since then I have discovered that I don't feel threatened by adversarial, menacing people, that I am more tolerant of distant, emotionally unavailable people, and that I am no longer concerned about my blue eyes! I benefited by staying in the understanding mode, or in this case more accurately, later returning to the understanding mode after having inadvertently immersed myself in my conflict. None of this would have happened if I had only immersed myself in my angry, hurt feelings about "ugly blue eyes," maligned the other guy whom I identified as the cause of my unrest, and walked off without my personal integrity.

Part 4: The importance of active understanding in raising children

Young children experience plenty of frustration and subsequent anger. Just watch one even under the best conditions. The amount of anger stimulated by the environment and how the child learns to handle it are of the utmost importance. A child who comes from an environment of much frustration and little tolerance for irritation will probably have lots of repressed anger and little ability to handle it other than with primitive, maladaptive techniques such as avoidance, denial, repression, or outright discharge of rage not only verbally but even physically. This child may have trouble learning in school and perform antisocial acts, eventually getting into trouble with the law. On the other hand, a child raised by evolved parents will have less frustration, less anger, and probably have learned to be comfortable with any fury they experience. They have likely learned to understand and accept these feelings, to identify and resolve conflicts which generate them, and to thereby reduce the amount of anger that might be in their lives. Because of this, they are probably freer, calmer, more able to focus, concentrate, and learn in school and have all of their energies available for study, play or enjoyment. They will have fewer feelings that seek discharge in antisocial ways.

Obviously, the quality of early childhood is critical. This was shown in an early 1990s New York study where the first four years of a child's life were rated with respect to quality of upbringing and later to the child's adjustment to society and performance in the classroom. There was a remarkably positive correlation between poor childhood-raising and subsequent poor social adjustment, leading to school dropouts and hostile antisocial behavior resulting in arrests. Learning to handle our emotions is like learning to coordinate our physical selves; for example, learning to walk: we go from uncertainty and awkwardness to coordination and skill. Just as parents will teach a child to walk, it is critical for the developing child, as well as society, for parents to provide a facilitative emotional environment.

The evolution of a human being is very complicated. Under optimal conditions we would, from early childhood, grow to acquire a level of comfort with ourselves, with the expression of our opinions, with an ability to easily enjoy ourselves, and with a relaxed means of perceiving and dealing with the world and its occupants. Hopefully, all of this unfolds unimpeded. When it doesn't, it is because something blocked it. For example, a child is frequently criticized by others for expressing their honest opinion. This hurts the child, who now may become reluctant to risk putting forth their view of things. Being so shut-up is too restrictive. Eventually, the child will try again to risk expression of their perceptions in an effort to overcome their fear of criticism. In doing so, if left to their own devices, they will seek out competitive, rejecting, even hostile relationships like the original ones that overwhelmed them emotionally. If they can't find, provoke, or create a restrictive relationship, they may imagine and experience it even if the listener is entirely comfortable and receptive to what they have to say. It is as if they must re-confront the dragon; go back to where they got overwhelmed and this time, somehow come out on top. In slightly other terms, they go back to where their evolution was stopped and attempt to go from there.

Aside from a few early appearing childhood maladies such as attention deficit disorder, hyperactivity syndromes, autism, etc., the average child only presents its parents/caretakers with a wide range of understandable totally childish behaviors. Given this, at these times it is hoped that parents welcome the opportunity to assist their kids. However, parental/caretaker responses range from being comfortable to outraged. Those who stay in the understanding mode provide the most facilitative nurturing for their children.

Here is a very simple example of how understanding and being comfortable facilitate a healthy parent/child relationship. It is suppertime, the child is playing in the yard, and it's time to summon them. Keep in mind how often the child experiences the parent as nagging, has difficulty withdrawing him or herself from whatever they're involved in, and appears to resist the parent. To create understanding, the parent should pause for just a moment to consider what the emotional task of withdrawal from a particular activity will require of the child; *then* ask the child to come in without making any effort to use new phraseology. Even this simple pause will make it easier for them. You will be surprised to discover that they come in easily and promptly just because of the new understanding and appreciation reflected in the parent's different manner of calling them in. It is not necessary for the parent to say "I know that you are very involved in your activity and withdrawing from that will not be easy, but supper is on the table, and we are ready to sit down, and you need to come in right now." Just this little *inner empathic understanding* and appreciation of the child will have somehow been communicated by the altered timing or tone of voice. As I said, this is a very simple example. But it can be very effective and it is something that you can teach yourself simply by pausing to think and using what you already know about people. It is simply the application of active understanding.

The most competent parents are comfortable with their children at all times. This is because they understand not only the children but themselves. If a child is able to hurt, annoy or upset the parent, a number of unfortunate things occur.

- First, the parent emotionally withdraws and the child is temporarily without a competent parent.
- Second, the child feels bad about themselves because they hurt the parent.
- Third, to whatever extent the child's mean, ornery, or angry wish existed, it was gratified and its discharge via hostile channels was encouraged.
- Fourth, the child, who cannot yet control himself, that is, avoid repeating the above upset, is without help and becomes fixated at this level. Because of this, both the child's inner and outer worlds become dangerous or chaotic.

Ideally, a child can bring the most primitive and troublesome aspects of themselves into a relationship with a competent, comfortable understanding parent and resolve them. This occurs when the parent is not available to gratify any of the child's hostile wishes but only gratifies those that are not hostile and are characterized by some mutuality. If this does not happen the child will not evolve; he or she will become accustomed to discharging his or her anger directly through sadistic channels upon others. This becomes a liability for the child, who now has trouble trusting themselves in social situations, given their tendency to vent their anger directly. Now, much of the child's attention must be directed toward controlling their anger and avoiding situations that might evoke their anger. And this now becomes an extra burden and a source of uneasiness and low self-esteem.

Let's look at an example in which the troublesome parts of the child are resolved with the help of a parent. This example takes place in the physical arena, as opposed to all the previous examples which were verbal. I think it makes explicit, albeit in physical terms, some of the needs of a young child and how a parent must help them evolve emotionally. Here, in the physical arena, the parents, usually the father, are so much bigger and stronger as to be in a position to keep the child from causing any harm.

Five-year-old "Johnny" is a normal kid in every way. He looks forward to twenty minutes or so of roughhousing with his father, "Frank", every night before supper until Johnny becomes exhausted. Recently, Johnny has shown an increase in "exuberance" characterized by attempting to hit, kick, tackle, and knock down his father. Frank is very comfortable with this and welcomes the opportunity to accommodate these expressions. At the same time, Frank is careful not to provoke any of this as he only wants to deal with that which naturally and normally lies within Johnny and only with what Johnny chooses to express or let happen. Frank knows that if Johnny can bring his most primitive feelings into his relationship with him then he can help Johnny work them out. Frank looks upon this time with Johnny as absolutely crucial for Johnny's emotional growth. Johnny's most troublesome feelings may include everything from exuberance, greed, competitiveness, excitement, anger, mischief and murderous rage and just to make sure we've included everything, let's add "piss and vinegar."

Frank wants all of Johnny's emotional energy to someday be available to him and not locked in repression because it is associated with hostile impulses or other means of asocial expression. Frank is available to accept all of Johnny's impulses but will not gratify any of his sadistic ones by allowing Johnny to hurt him. This way, all of Johnny's energy can be made available to Johnny because it will not become fused or fixated in sadistic expression. The energy fueling his hostility remains alive and available to him for channels of more mutual expression. The energy does not become a liability as it would if it were fused with discharge via asocial channels. In fact, Johnny's sadistic impulses will be totally frustrated, that is, ungratified because his father is not hurt or made uncomfortable at all. Theoretically then, all of Johnny's emotional energy will be available to him and none will have to be repressed because it is associated with expression in hostile, sadistic ways.

So, Johnny and Frank roughhouse on the rug before supper almost every night. Frank is much bigger and stronger than Johnny and easily fends off his attacks so that no damage is done. During Johnny's more vicious moments, Frank has a comfortable twinkle in his eye and perhaps the proud thought that "*if this kid's out to kill his father at age five, he's ambitious and going somewhere in life. His energies just need a little channeling."* It goes without saying that failure to frustrate Johnny's most murderous impulses would not be good for Johnny or his father. In any event, as time passes, Johnny's emotional energy begins to go into impulses associated with more mutuality and less hostility. Johnny might say such things as "Dad, let's you and me play checkers" in a fairly aggressive manner and adding trustfully "but you help me too."

Johnny may also engage Frank in playing catch with a baseball, a fairly mutual activity, but only occasionally try to burn the palm of his father's hand! As Johnny grows up he can feel comfortable with himself because he could bring the most troublesome and vicious aspects of himself into the relationship with his father where there was no gratification of these hostile impulses, and, hence, no dangerous, destructive, *or "bad" parts of himself.* Johnny's energies do not have to be repressed and unavailable to him because they find gratification through antisocial outlets. His energies remain free and available for him to use comfortably wherever he chooses. And this will be accompanied by an increase in confidence and self-esteem in all parts of his life.

The essence of the above in terms of active understanding is that Johnny's anger, in the form of hostile physical acts, was *accepted* but not *gratified.* Frank was, in essence, saying *"Johnny, I can accept comfortably the fact that you have some wishes to hurt me. The important thing is that we acknowledge these wishes (through roughhousing) without gratifying them, that is, I will not allow you to hurt me. Our roughhousing is acceptable because I am bigger and stronger than you are and I can ensure both of our safety."*

In addition to the acknowledgment of these primitive impulses, Johnny also benefits by learning to forgo their expression until the designated roughhouse period. Here, as he is learning how to control them, he finds he no longer has to fear the loss of control. Moreover, at the same time, he has a chance to begin to identify and accept his anger. This lends itself to identifying his unrealistic expectations and recalibrating them. In short, his anger becomes a comfortable and recognizable signal that he has some unrealistic expectations that need his personal attention. While anger in the physical arena has real hazards for adults, it does have a place for small children who can be easily managed by their much bigger parents. In addition, we should be aware that small children may not yet be verbally articulate and are therefore better able to use a physical means of expression.

Obviously, not all children or all parents will find it suitable to work things out as Johnny and Frank did. And girls may have different ways of expressing themselves. Some children may do this simply over a checkerboard with their parents. Hopefully, the child will be able to risk bringing the most troublesome parts of themselves into a safe understanding relationship with a parent in some form where the expression of all impulses is accepted but where the hostile ones are not gratified. If the child can ever hurt the parent or have their hostile expression gratified, then they are "bad", they begin to savor sadistic means of discharge of their energies, to develop a negative self-image and become uncomfortable with their own anger. If the child, in trying to be "bad", is unable to hurt the parent no matter how hard they try, they can only conclude that they are not "bad" and go on to develop a positive image of themselves because *"if*

I brought the worst of me into the relationship with my dad and no damage was done, there can't be any part of me that's 'bad'."

Often children who are struggling with feeling wrong about themselves turn to their parents for help through some sort of provocation and find their worst fears confirmed. This is because the parent takes it personally, is preoccupied with making sure the child's behavior conforms to their standards, or is just "busy" and not available to employ the active understanding approach. For example, if a child does something blatantly selfish, it may be that they themselves are feeling selfish and want to make an issue of it. Or, it could be that they feel deprived and are trying to revoke some compensation. Or, it could be that they are experimenting with what they perceive to be an adult prerogative. In any event, hopefully, the parent can bring their comfort and interest in understanding to the child and see what happens. When the child finds the parent helpful in dealing with their problems they can discard the provocations. And, eventually they can use what they learned from their parents to resolve their conflicts by themselves.

Here is an example from my own life. I took my two-and-a half-year-old grandson to the local airport to watch the planes take off and land. On the way back to the car, I arrived first and opened the passenger door for him, only to discover that he had stopped about thirty feet away on the sidewalk. He had a very uncomfortable look on his face. It then occurred to me that he was being obstreperous by not following me to the car. My immediate response was to let him know that I was entirely comfortable with him and with whatever he was about. I tried to convey this by saying nothing, just looking at him with calm and patience. I did not give him permission to delay; this is something he's working out with himself and requires more time. Experimenting with noncompliance is quite appropriate for a child in their "terrible twos", often characterized by "no" or "I won't." Today it resulted in our being delayed no more than two minutes. While nothing more became of this in our relationship, his working out his noncompliance remains acceptable and available for understanding. If I had been uncomfortable or irate with his experimentation, then he would be less free to experiment with, understand, and accept this part of himself. Again, I simply showed him I was comfortable with his behavior and did not give him permission to delay in order to work out being negative or obstinate.

It is unrealistic to expect children, even your children, not to have some primitive, unmodified, unrecognized, mean impulses. They will have sadistic urges – the trick is to not gratify them by allowing them to affect you, that is, their attempts to annoy or hurt you are completely frustrated. This way, their sadistic modes of expression will gradually disappear because there is no means of gratification. Their energy will begin to find expression through more socially acceptable channels because that is all that is available for gratification of their desires. This way all of their emotional energy remains available to them rather than becoming a liability associated with sadistic expression.

Here's another example: "Steve," a divorced father and his girlfriend "Heather" went skiing up in the mountains. They brought along his preadolescent son "Kevin" and two of his friends from school. As they drove up to the mountains the young boys seated in the back of the car tried to be as obnoxious as possible with outrageous behavior. They talked roughly, swearing at every opportunity, and passed gas as loudly as they could. They were clearly trying out some new behavior. Perhaps they aspired to become world experts in offensive teenage behavior, who knows? Steve and Heather were comfortable enough with the whole thing, actually sort of amused by it and curious as to how it might fare. This behavior continued into the second or third day when in the afternoon after skiing, Kevin approached Heather on the stairs as she was taking a bottle of champagne to the master bedroom. Kevin said to her in an impromptu, spontaneous, and as insufferable-as-he-could way, "I'll bet my dad's going to pump you dry." Heather paused, looked him squarely in the eye, and said "By gosh he'd better!" and proceeded up the stairs. At this point there was an amazing change in all the boys' behavior. Their talk became extremely polite and considerate. They could not do enough for her, holding her chair, offering to fetch things for her, etc. They treated her like a queen. This continued throughout the remainder of the trip to the amusement of both Steve and Heather.

Here, the preadolescent boys were experimenting with outrageous behavior. It contained an obviously hostile element. The ski trip could accommodate their conduct and the adults were comfortable with it and the aggression. Given this, no damage was done to either party; the adults were not made uneasy or harmed and the boys' potentially antagonistic attempts were not gratified. Gratifying them would actually be harmful to the boys, fixating their sadistic desires. The turning point appears to have been when the boys could not make the adults, particularly Heather, uncomfortable with their utmost blatant aggression. Here, Steve and Heather did not supply the masochistic complement for the boys attempted sadism to the extent that it may actually have existed. The boys were completely frustrated with respect to their attempts (sadistic drives) to upset the adults. Given this, the boys' behavior took a dramatic shift to mutuality, actually beyond mutuality, the boys championed her! Had they been successful in teasing the adults, a gratification of their sadistic impulses, this transition would not have occurred.

Here is a very subtle example. See if you can pick up the child's conflict and how you might help her with it. On a birthday card nicely decorated with stars, a nine-year-old girl wrote to her mother, *"Dear mom, you have to know that I love you, brother, and dad more than anything in the whole wide world. I designed your card like this because you are a STAR mom and the only thing I'd like to say right now is I love you and happy birthday!!! You are always smiling and/or happy. You take great care of us and love us all. Whenever I get mad or say something bad to you I NEVER mean it. I am very lucky of having you as my mom. You are THE BEST mom in the whole world. Love, your daughter Patricia."*

The sentence *"whenever I get mad or say something bad to you I never mean it"* suggests that she cannot accept her anger or her previous expressions of it. This means that there is a part of her emotional self that she cannot accept. Her anger is real, she is aware of it, and fortunately, she has been able to *acknowledge* it. Moreover, she has been able to bring this troubled part of herself into her relationship with her mother, which should be the safest, most trusted, and hopefully most facilitative relationship available to her. In short, she has certainly done her part by bringing her real self, for better or worse, into her relationship with mom. However, she has trouble *accepting* her anger and could use any help that her mother might have available.

Recognizing this, how can we help her? We could begin to watch for her irritations, try to understand them, and make our comfort with them available to her emotionally during these times. This would invite her to bring these feelings into her relationship with us where she can borrow on our understanding and ease with her distress and its source. In her evolution as a child, her anger will probably be perceived initially as a result of her parents not supplying her immediate needs (when you think about raising children, this is not a very profound statement!) Hopefully, whenever the child experiences anger, it can be comfortably accepted by the parents. Once this happens, then our attention can be directed to its source. If the anger is not accepted comfortably, the chances of ever getting to its source are greatly reduced. Therefore, whenever anger appears, a premium must be placed upon it.

- First, we accept their anger–we are very interested in it and invite them to talk about it.
- Then, we look for the source of it–we get them to fully explore what they blame their anger upon. This may take the form of first projecting the blame upon us, discovering that we are comfortable with this possibility and then acquiring a new level of comfort with their projection so that they can accept it as their own and begin to process it appropriately.

This is accomplished by our profound comfort, understanding, acceptance, and interest in anger. Hopefully, all and any household anger will automatically be dealt with in this way.

Your expressed interest alone in your child's distress will be appreciated by him as all children need help mastering their anger by accepting it, especially by putting it into words, and then aligning their expectations realistically with the world. Hopefully, in the beginning their anger can be accepted in whatever form it presents itself. In a young child the expression may first be physical. Gentle restraint may be necessary. We never allow them to hurt us with their anger because we are physically much bigger and because we are so comfortable with all of their feelings. Hopefully, our interest and receptiveness to their emotions will invite them to focus on their anger and begin to talk about it. As they explore it, they can begin to see how reasonable or unreasonable it is. However, even if the child's anger is over an entirely unrealistic wish, the examination of the wish with them is crucial.

How often do we hear "have you been a good or a bad child today?" Here, the child has a chance to begin to view a part of themselves as unacceptable, or "bad," and to be avoided, and therefore, not subject to understanding. It's also an invitation to devoting their life to meeting their parents' standards rather than developing their own personal integrity, that is, *"I exist to please my parents."* Hopefully, as parents, rather than asking if they have been good or bad, we will ask them about what they enjoyed, what they may have mastered in their lives, what new things they learned today, did they win or lose and how did they feel about it.

Likewise, in punishing a child, it is destructive to make them feel bad about their very being, that is, *"you are a bad person."* At times a child may require punishing but it should be done for their behavior and not because their being is "bad." For example, a child may deliberately break the rules or do something unsafe in order to explore or test the consequences, which are actually just learning about certain aspects of reality. This doesn't mean that the child's *being* is "bad." The negative reinforcement, the punishment, should be associated with the dangerous and undesirable behavior, such as stepping off the curb. In the adult world it's a little bit like a speeding ticket in which a particular behavior, speeding, may evoke negative reinforcement in the form of a traffic ticket. Here, it doesn't mean that our beings are bad; it just means that we engaged in behavior that resulted in a penalty.

Parents who successfully incorporate active understanding into their relationships with their children are giving them a strong foundation that will set them on a course to healthy adult relationships, instill in them the ability to acknowledge and accept anger, and allow them to grow into personalities with integrity.

Part 5: How active understanding impacts our relationships

Earlier we discussed the thrust to grow that exists in all of us. The success of this *thrust to grow emotionally is greatly enhanced by another's understanding and comfort level with it.* This comfort level comes from their awareness and understanding of what the person attempting to grow emotionally is about. And it can be obtained simply by an active understanding approach in any and all relationships where a premium is placed upon accepting and understanding anger. It is surprisingly easily obtained by simply practicing attempting to understand anger and adversity with our own humanness; we just need to give our humanness a chance by staying in the understanding mode a few more seconds and discovering how often the situation is eased when we do. Most, if not all of us possess the capacity to do this but too often we don't take the time to attempt the kind of understanding necessary to realize it. When we do, we invite ourselves to grow emotionally and are better able to maintain our integrity and stay in the external here-and-now rather than regress within ourselves.

In any relationship, if we observe and understand exactly what is going on with the other person, we can best accept it for exactly what it is: reality. Even if there are disappointments in the relationship, rejection or anger, our understanding helps to make it okay *because it is just reality*. When we don't understand and accept disappointment, rejection or anger, our ability to adapt is compromised. The understanding approach connects us to reality which we can then comprehend, accept and utilize adaptively. The acceptance of reality is meaningful, safe, reliable and always accompanied by a sense of satisfaction: *"this is okay because it's what reality is providing for today."* This sense of satisfaction is achieved because we are at one with ourselves and the world. This can only come about by an active understanding and acceptance of our feelings, our perceptions/misperceptions, and ourselves. Not until we have achieved this can the environment (reality) become something that we can assess without distortion or manipulation for our emotional needs. It not only feels good to be at one with reality, it is safe and adaptive. It helps us avoid the narcissistic defaults that plague our lives and allows us to live with personal integrity.

When it comes to interpersonal relationships, ideally our decision to be around somebody is based on mutual appreciation of accurate appraisal and not love. This is because the greatest enjoyment and gratification of a relationship come from connecting with the reality of that person: what they have to say, their reactions to themselves, us, and the world; their style of doing things, the fun we can have with them, what they're willing to risk, what they expect from us, their comfort with us, their creativity, and, last but not least, their personal integrity. This is an alternative to "love" which is really a feeling or quality we have projected upon them stemming from our own ungratified wishes, even though, admittedly, it often just feels good!

Likewise, hopefully, our decision *not* to be around somebody is based on understanding and not upon anger or damnation of their being. In this case, if we elect not to be around someone based on understanding, it means that we can comfortably accept them but simply choose not to do so because of our preferences. Amazingly, when understanding another we think we don't "like", they often become more interesting. If we choose not to be with them because of our anger, it means that we have not resolved our associated conflicts, which we are probably now mismanaging by blaming, avoiding, and or maligning them. We have left reality and are not making a choice from our personal integrity.

Understanding reality increases our ability to adapt. We can increase our ability to perceive and understand external reality (the world beyond ourselves) by ridding ourselves of emotional conflicts that interfere with our perception of reality and our understanding of it. In human beings, it appears that our feelings (emotions) most commonly provide this interference.

We must apply and maintain *active understanding* of what we can observe, and be wary of emotional states that can interfere with our observations and with their interpretations. Instead of responding with discomfort, withdrawing within a troubled part of ourselves, and/or maligning others, we can now avoid all of this with our understanding and stay connected to them with a comfortable receptivity. Practically, this means that any problem or conflict brought into the verbal arena will be subjected to listening, understanding, a level of comfort, and thus invited in the direction of resolution. Here, we could all grow emotionally, find security in relationships, and develop more real and meaningful connections with our fellow citizens. This means that help is available for any troubled person just by bringing their anger into the verbal arena. Just think how this would empower society and bring a new mutuality among us.

Hopefully, you feel ready to employ an active understanding approach in your relationships and with your own unresolved issues. Play around with it and you will discover how adept you can become by staying in the understanding mode just a few seconds longer in difficult situations, or, in situations that you previously found difficult. You may find that much of psychology can be very self-evident.

Chapter 4:

———•◦•———

How Personal Integrity & Active Understanding Help Society

We have seen the importance of understanding and acceptance of our troublesome feelings: the reality of ourselves. When we understand and accept, we may be able to resolve our emotional conflicts and evolve our personalities. Once we have done this we are in a better position to accurately perceive and process external reality and to become "at one" with it, which is a very soothing and satisfying experience. In short, the more we can accept the reality of ourselves, the greater our chances of accurately perceiving and optimally dealing with external reality.

Raising Children

In raising our children, we would become adept at assessing their needs and meeting them as appropriate rather than letting our unresolved issues interfere. This would mean that we understand them as entities developing their own personal integrity and do not view them as extensions of ourselves. We should not use them as vehicles for demonstrating what wonderful parents we are. Whatever behavior they present to us would first be subjected to an active understanding of not only what it represents in terms of their personality growth but also which of their wishes should be gratified and which ones should not be gratified. While at times their behavior may be unacceptable, at no time would they be deemed "bad" as this would mean that their very being is unacceptable and must be avoided. Actually and most amazingly, just having an awareness of the child's real needs (an aspect of reality) often provides all the motivation we need to meet them. And when one gratifies their child's real and appropriate needs parenthood becomes as satisfying as it can get! Not all of our children's wishes are to be gratified but we always accept their wishes with understanding and are delighted to be their parent.

Politics

So many politicians appear to be unable to discern the overall needs of the country, apparently because they can't get beyond their personal idealisms, their party's politics, and/or their need for re-election. These are, in my opinion, all narcissistic defaults. With active understanding, theoretically at least, even politicians would be able to get beyond their personal idealism and party politics to understand the overall needs of the country and work to affect their implementation. Here's my image of an ideal politician:

A campaigning politician says to a smiling, affable, wanting-to-bond guy whom he's never met who wants to shake his hand,

"I'm not interested in your vote. I don't want to shake your hand. I don't want to pretend we're buddies. I don't care if you like me. I think I have something worth your while to understand. I want to present it to all for your consideration. If you find it helpful, apply it to your voting, and vote for whomever you think will best implement it. Again, I'm not here to try to get your vote or to cater to your whims. I'm here to present my understanding as best I can and comfortably accept wherever the voting process takes us. I don't know if what I have to bring is helpful at all. And, I don't even know if you have the capacity to determine if it's helpful. Actually, I doubt that you do because you invited me to enter into a relationship with you based on artificiality." I like to think that this politician has integrity and is not at the voters' beck and call.

Social Issues

The mindless application of our ideals to society's problems because it makes us feel better about ourselves to do so, is a self-serving, or narcissistic, default. The simplistic application of ideals requires no thinking or understanding. "Tough decisions" will have to be made and this can only be done with active understanding. Here are some examples:

- We give citizenship to an illegal alien because we feel everybody deserves what we have in this country. This is done solely for our needs; to make us feel better, more righteous. Instead, we could begin to assess the problematic situation of immigration realistically and plan an appropriate and facilitative solution based on understanding and not on our desire to feel good about ourselves. In this situation, if we consider the motivation of people who are so dissatisfied with the economic and social conditions in their countries of origin that they come here, perhaps giving them a work visa and returning them to their home country where they might agitate for change and eventually give millions of people in their country of origin a taste of what we have here, would be a better long term solution. This example shows how easily one's narcissistic needs to feel good about themselves by using the environment could penalize a lot of people!

- "All men are created equal" is often mindlessly offered as a solution to problems in order to be "fair" so we can feel good about ourselves and avoid dealing with understanding the problems created by the fact that people have grossly different needs and abilities.

- We capture a member of a terrorist sect who is twelve hours away from detonating a nuclear bomb in Manhattan that would kill millions of people. Our inclination is to insist upon reading him his Miranda rights and helping him get a lawyer in order to "maintain our principles" of freedom, again so we can feel good about ourselves. An appraisal of the situation of the terrorist and his sect would determine if we really do have such a luxury and would have nothing to do with a disregard for freedom.

- "Going green" has become an ideal for some people. They feel better, for example, advocating the production of ethanol for automobiles despite the fact that almost as much energy is required to produce the ethanol as it will provide. And using corn for this purpose keeps the price of it up so high that starving populations in other countries dependent upon corn can no longer afford to buy it. Hopefully, our "going green" will be based on more realistic active understanding in which our intent is upon meeting the restorative needs or requirements of a problem regardless of the outcome and not based on our use of the environment to make ourselves feel better. Our dealing with the reality of the problem can be plenty interesting enough.

These are just a few of the narcissistic defaults that I believe occur in the absence of active understanding. I like to think that staying in reality with active understanding leads to narcissistic defaults simply fading out.

We tend to view society as our creation and, therefore, think it is receptive to our ideals. But society is not. It is a part of nature and subject to the laws of nature and, therefore, must be approached with active understanding. It is my opinion that we have reached a time in history where our survival will be dependent upon our understanding instead of the mindless application of ideals.

While getting beyond yourself and staying in the here-and-now external reality with the understanding approach will probably be practiced mostly in interpersonal situations, it certainly has application in understanding and dealing with social and worldly issues. Besides nuclear bombs and terrorists, we are confronted by a waning middle class, questions about whom to tax and how much, a high percentage of high school dropouts, too many citizens who cannot support a democracy, unsustainable entitlements, most of the wealth in the hands of a very few, to name just a few of our current issues. Hopefully, our understanding of these problems can dictate our actions and we will not just throw money at them, apply an unrealistic idealism, subject them to political goals, or neglect them entirely.

Incarceration

With respect to our treatment of convicted criminals, an understanding approach to their thrusts to grow and evolve themselves offers more with respect to rehabilitation than a punishment for their antisocial behavior. As we have seen, declaring somebody "bad" or "evil" and then deciding how much to punish them has little to do with reality. This is not to say that certain behaviors should not warrant negative reinforcement or incarceration but this is for their *act* and not for their *being*.

Psychiatry

Given my years as a psychotherapist, I can't close this book without a psychiatric comment. While I have treated only a few patients in intensive psychotherapy (two or more times a week over a period of years) who were diagnosed with schizophrenia, I have come to believe that evolving their personality by resolving emotional conflicts in intensive long-term psychotherapy is effective in helping them achieve a happier life and a permanent disappearance of all psychotic symptoms. This was achieved with only a few patients with whom I got to work intensively over an extended period of time.

The following metaphor demonstrates the relationship between sound adaptation in reality and the defaults. A child has a scooter which he or she rides by standing with one foot on the scooter, pushing with the other foot to get going, and then coasting for a while standing on both feet. The child is not yet very skillful at riding the scooter and often falls. Children with a short right leg often fall to the right and children with a short left leg often fall to the left. Here, the default is determined by their nature (genes).

Rather than refer to falling to the right as "right leg syndrome," or referring to falling to the left as "left leg disease," it makes more sense to focus on the child's ability, or inability, to ride the scooter. If we help the child to become more adept at riding the scooter through instruction and practice then they will stop falling. Too often we focus our attention and/ or treatment on a default, dignifying it with a diagnosis or labeling it as a "syndrome" instead of focusing on the primary problem. This is not to say that identification and resolution of the primary problem will be easy, it will take a great deal of active understanding and effort.

In light of the above, it is my opinion that the major psychiatric diagnoses can, in some way, be viewed as genetically determined defaults to which the patient turns during periods of emotional integration failure. The penetration of these various genetic predispositions varies considerably, from profound to weak. Likewise, people's emotional integrative capacities vary considerably, from reliable to capricious. This active understanding approach to the treatment of psychotic disorders would be in addition to the common one of prescribing anti-psychotic drugs. At times, the judicious use of anti-psychotic drugs may be necessary to keep patients functioning, working, or in on-going psychotherapy. Hopefully, the patient will participate in the decision to use them. It is my hope that a little more consideration will be given to the advantages of the evolving patient and the use of active understanding in psychotherapy rather than just focusing on symptoms. For example, help the paranoid to accept their projections, the depressed to accept their disappointments and anger, or the anxious to accept their uncomfortable impulses.

In conclusion

I believe that there is an inherent drive in all of us to evolve. This may not only take the form of mastering troublesome parts of ourselves by identifying, understanding, accepting, and resolving, but of doing the same thing with problems of humanity in the external world. I like to think that when we really understand and accept reality we will find that it virtually dictates what we should do for the best interests of ourselves and humanity. For example, if we see starving, homeless, hurting, stagnating, sad, wayward people, the mere reality of this would have a mind with integrity wondering how to help fix it and attempt to do so depending upon their means and availability. We would do this primarily because we want to meet the realistic needs of these people, addressing and responding to the mere reality of it is rewarding enough. This would be quite different from simply trying to make these people feel better because that makes us feel better. Although I know little about Bill Gates or Warren Buffet and their philanthropy, I am impressed that they appear to have gotten beyond themselves, discerned some of the problems of the world, and set out to fix them.

Here, I think, is another example of one getting beyond themselves rather than using the environment to meet their emotional needs. In an interview with Judy Woodruff, the astronaut John Glenn was asked, "In fact, Senator, you are seen as an American hero for what you did. What does that mean to you?" He replied, "Well, to me, I leave those observations up to other people. I don't look at myself that way. I can guarantee you that..."

Let's look at one last example where a little active understanding and maintaining personal integrity could have gone a long way. I heard a story about a man who gave a $2 million birthday party for his wife. The venue was very special, the decorations elaborate, and the entertainment famous and from afar. I assumed the man, and perhaps his wife, were using the environment to meet their emotional needs of self-aggrandizement. My next thought was that with their awareness of the housing situation, the large number of underwater mortgages, and the high percentage of families that will lose their homes, they might have thought "the greatest birthday satisfaction" could come from using that $2 million to keep twenty families from being thrown out of their homes (might be structured in such a way that most of the $2 million would eventually be recovered) and enjoying the meaningful and rewarding interpersonal connections that a $50,000 birthday party would prompt. Here, at least in my opinion, the environment was used to meet their emotional needs which precluded a response to the reality of the real external world and the gratification that can come from it.

Our first step to live with integrity is that we must be able to accept the reality of ourselves through understanding all of our needs and feelings, particularly our anger as a signal. It all starts here. Once we can do this, we can get beyond ourselves and accurately perceive and process external reality. Otherwise, we approach the external environment for the purpose of fulfilling our needs stemming from our troubled emotions, which limits our ability to accurately perceive reality and our ability to become "at one" with it, a rewarding and satisfying experience. It may be that the appeal of meditation is precisely this, that is, connecting to reality per se is so satisfying and restorative.

When we don't take another's expression of anger at us personally, it is thanks to our personal integrity. This benefits us because we avoid the narcissistic defaults that keep us out of external reality. It also benefits the other, the aggressor, because it nullifies their attempts to hurt us, it keeps the relationship safe and it invites understanding. It is important to remember that our response, as helpful as it may have been to them, was entirely incidental to the preservation of our integrity and our staying in reality, and had nothing to do with our "giving or sacrificing of ourselves" for the other.

I'm not sure whether reality or integrity is the end in itself; maybe it's both, but I don't think you can have one without the other. Let your integrity and your awareness of reality (inner and outer) take you where it may. Good luck!

Acknowledgments

Thank you to my family, friends and all the people in my life who made this book possible. Special thanks to my editor Dena Fischer, publicist Andrea Burnett, cover art designer Airiel Mulvaney and my assistant Megan Hornbecker for all of their hard work and dedication. And lastly, thank you to the human race for inspiring me throughout my career and to write this book.

For more information on this book and to share how *Achieving Personal Integrity* has affected you, please visit:
www.achievingpersonalintegrity.com